2009

THE INSIDER'S GUIDE
TO
DEMENTIA CARE

What You Should Know About Assisted Living, Alzheimer's, And Dementia Care

KATHERINE E. GOETHE, PhD

and

MARTHA E. LEATHERMAN, MD

with

KATHLEEN O'BRIEN

WingSpan Press

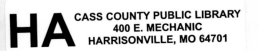

Printed in the United States of America

Published by WingSpan Press, Livermore, CA
www.wingspanpress.com

The WingSpan name, logo and colophon are the trademarks of WingSpan Publishing.

ISBN 978-1-59594-315-6
First edition 2009

Library of Congress Control Number 2009931462

CONTENTS

Introduction: From the Trenches
THE REALITY OF ASSISTED LIVING
AND LONG-TERM CARE

What, really, is the fear of growing old? Most people say, "Being lonely," "Being neglected," or "Being in pain." We all have seen those pitiful images of warehoused elderly lined up in wheelchairs against an institutional wall. When one considers that an entire generation of elders has been allowed to age this way, there is guilt and grief at the same time. In response to the dawning horror at the dehumanization of people in long term care, efforts were spawned to establish independent living, assisted living, and the concept of "aging in place." Despite this remarkable expansion in options available to elders needing assistance, the nagging fear of "placement" in any facility remains. Why? Because we all recognize the unfortunate reality that even with the improvements in long-term care, most retirement facilities are still woefully inadequate in providing the most fundamental understanding, love, and real emotional caring that are essential to anyone's quality of life and dignity. The inadequacy is most obvious in the case of elders with dementia.

As specialists in the psychiatric and psychological complications of aging, we have spent the greater part of our careers caring for those ravaged by the chronic pain and mental illnesses associated with aging: most prominently the many forms of dementia (including Alzheimer's), depression, and delirium. On the frontlines of geriatric health care, we have seen all too clearly how not to care for the aged, and we have been shocked to realize how little the elder care industry really knows about the brain diseases affecting older people. This recognition came to a head after we were contacted by a prestigious long-term care facility for help in setting up a separate Alzheimer's/dementia unit. We discovered that no fundamental base of knowledge was even required to establish and market a dementia care unit, and there were no real standards for specialized training programs in behavioral modification for aides and nurses working in such units. Even training of staff in non-dementia care facilities was hit or miss.

We knew that psychologists, physicians, and nurses had to undergo rigorous training and testing for certification in order to treat patients. We had previously assumed that there were educational institutions that had courses and certification procedures to ensure that caretakers in assisted living and long-term care facilities had special training for the provision of optimal dementia care. Instead, we were disturbed to find that each facility had its own, individual in-house training program which varied widely from one facility to another. Maybe the staff would attend occasional lectures presented by the Alzheimer's Association, maybe not. At that time, there was no central place, no educational institution, and no curriculum that provided specialized training for caretakers in assisted living and long-term care facilities.

Believing that the state (in our case, Texas) had oversight of the certification process for assisted living and long-term health care workers, we looked up the state regulations, which mandate the amount of training required for direct-care staff (i.e., nurses, nurses' aides, medication aides) in assisted living and long-term care facilities and dementia care units. We discovered that training requirements were sorely lacking. Since that time, the hours of required training have increased over the years, with a menu of topics provided. Additionally, there are requirements for annual continuing education, but unlike other health care workers such as nurses, there is no credentialing agency to determine the adequacy of training for aides working in assisted living and long-term care facilities and dementia units. Even more disturbing is the fact that regulations and standards also vary from state to state. Some states have no regulations or standards at all.

When continuing education is provided by facilities, we have observed that the opportunities to teach and to create a high-quality learning experience are dismal. During 30-minute or 1-hour educational sessions (called "in-services"), attendees come and go, sleep, do paperwork, or look at their watches. Some make eye contact or nod their heads as we talk, but at the end of the training session, they all quickly scatter without any questions or comments. We know because we've taught and observed these "continuing education" courses.

After seeing all these problems, we decided there had to be a better way to disseminate information and to educate dementia caregivers in assisted living and long-term care facilities. There had to be dignity for the person with dementia, dignity for family members— and dignity for professional caregivers. New aides who received inadequate training were certainly not being afforded much dignity. It was not the aides' fault—they could only provide care at the level they had been taught. So, we founded Dignity First® as an entity dedicated to providing a structured program of training in dementia and aging.

This book was born of our frustrating experiences as we tried to provide consulting services to residents of long term care facilities and, through Dignity First®, tried to offer our ideas and training to the administrators and owners of facilities. It seemed logical to us that our training programs would be the solution to an increasing need, since we are considered the experts called in by assisted living and long-term care facilities whenever they encounter obstacles in caring for a resident with dementia.

After months, we grew weary of the enthusiastic and friendly initial reactions to our goals, followed by the lack of understanding of what we were trying to accomplish and the inevitable roadblock of cost-cutting, no matter the real cost to the long-term care facility's residents by denying them the best available care. We have heard all the excuses for not providing adequate training: the budgetary priority of new uniforms or new lobby furniture, the false confidence in existing training methods, the outright denial that more training is necessary, the denial that assisted living residents have any evidence of dementia, *ad infinitum*. Even more disturbing was the lack of concern about the effect that inadequate training had on the residents and their families. Frustrated families did not know where to turn, were afraid to complain, and would ask us to intervene for them. Unfortunately, even our "expert" voices went unheeded.

We have all heard the statistics about the aging population, the increase in dementia, and the decreased numbers of nurses and caregivers. We must all do something about the crisis that is already here and growing more serious. Consumer advocacy groups are not enough. One good nurse in a facility is not enough. The financial bottom line is not enough. Governmental regulations are not enough. A fish tank at the nurse's station and attractive décor for mood elevation and a soothing environment are not enough. It's all been tried and, hopefully, you will come to the same conclusions we have: Without a foundation of knowledge and adequate professional, certified training in eldercare— and dementia care, in particular— the quality of life of residents in assisted living and long-term care facilities cannot be optimized. To deny adequate training to caregivers, we are not only hiding the problem, we are also hiding from the problem.

It has been said by industry leaders that assisted living is consumer-driven, and if consumers are unhappy with care, then they can move to another facility. Such dismissal of the real problems is shameful. We decided that if the industry really believes it is consumer-driven, then we needed to inform the consumers about how to drive the industry. This book provides solutions, options, choices, and, ultimately empowerment. Advocacy takes effort. Change takes effort. But we believe that families and residents in assisted living and dementia care are ready to take action.

Author Profiles

KATHERINE ELIZABETH GOETHE, PhD

Dr. Goethe is a psychologist who specializes in the neuropsychology of aging. In her independent private practice, she evaluates the elderly and counsels their families. In addition, she sees patients at the Neurology Center of San Antonio and evaluates residents in nursing homes, assisted living facilities, and retirement communities. She also leads a family support group for the Alzheimer's Association.

Dr. Goethe received her PhD in clinical psychology from Virginia Commonwealth University in 1983. She completed her residency training at the Medical University of South Carolina and completed two years of study in neuropsychology under the supervision of Dr. Harvey Levin at the University of Texas Medical Branch at Galveston. She and her husband live in San Antonio.

MARTHA E. LEATHERMAN, MD

Dr. Leatherman is a physician with specialty board certification in geriatric psychiatry and special expertise in geriatric mental health. She maintains a private practice, evaluating and treating elderly adults. She also performs competency evaluations for guardianship proceedings, and is an expert in the effects of undue influence.

Dr. Leatherman received her medical degree and

residency training in psychiatry from the University of Texas Medical School at Houston and completed a fellowship in the psychopharmacology and psychobiology of mood disorders at the University of North Carolina at Chapel Hill. She subsequently became a member of the faculty at the University of Texas Medical School at San Antonio. Dr. Leatherman has been recognized as an outstanding teacher and scientific investigator by organizations such as the Southern Association for Research in Psychiatry and the New Clinical Drug Evaluation Unit of the National Institute of Mental Health. She has authored and presented numerous peer-reviewed articles and is currently a much sought-after speaker for organizations such as Community Mental Health Centers, judicial organizations, assisted living facilities, and family support groups.

Dr. Leatherman lives outside San Antonio with her husband and children.

In 2003, Dr. Leatherman and Dr. Goethe established Dignity First®, dedicated to improving caregiver skills through high-quality interactive training seminars. The website for their organization is DignityFirst.net.

WITH EDITORIAL SUPPORT FROM KATHLEEN O'BRIEN

Kathleen O'Brien has a B.A. degree in English from Macalester College in St. Paul, Minnesota. She has had a long career in medical publishing, most of it with Little, Brown and Company, and is currently a freelance editor and writer. She, her husband, and son reside in San Antonio.

Acknowledgment

We wish to thank Kathy O'Brien for her assistance in making this book a reality. We are also very grateful to our husbands for their enduring support and encouragement. To the families who so willingly shared their stories we extend special thanks.

THE INSIDER'S GUIDE

TO

DEMENTIA CARE

CHAPTER ONE
An Introduction to Alzheimer's and the Brain

In this book there are many examples of the behavior problems that people with Alzheimer's disease, or other sorts of dementia, can have. These behavior problems can be made much worse when they are not properly managed by caregivers. In order for you to better understand the examples and the issues discussed, you first need some basic information about the brain and how a brain with dementia affects a person's behavior. Appendix B and Appendix C provide a much more detailed discussion of the brain, causes of dementia, how dementia is diagnosed, and brain functions. Those sections can be used as references to find out more information as you read through the book. For now, though, an introduction should be enough.

Strictly speaking, dementia is a very general term that describes disease processes in the brain that are marked by changes in behavior and thinking (cognition). Table 1 lists symptoms and behaviors associated with dementia. Not all of these behaviors need to be present in order to diagnose dementia, and not all of these are associated with every type of dementia. In addition, persons may exhibit some of these behaviors and not have dementia at all. Any and all of these symptoms can occur in a person in the later stages of Alzheimer's disease.

Table 1.
Symptoms and behaviors associated with dementia.

Memory loss
Repeated questions or statements
Difficulties doing everyday tasks (writing, handling money)
Loss of concentration
Tendency to lose things
Disorientation and getting lost in familiar places
Sundowning (restlessness/agitation in the evening)
Social withdrawal
Incontinence
Fear of bathing
Difficulties walking
Clumsiness
Speech difficulties
Confusion
Wandering
Difficulty following instructions
Seeing things that aren't there
Delusions/Bizarre ideas
Depression
Anger that is excessive or out of character
Violence
Paranoia
Cognitive fluctuations
Difficulty thinking
Apathy
Poor judgment
Compulsive behaviors, such as eating or hoarding
Inappropriate sexual behavior
Loss of recognition of familiar people

Alzheimer's disease is only one of the many forms of dementia, although it is the most common. Other than Alzheimer's, there are a number of types of dementia, such as vascular dementia, Lewy Body Dementia, frontotemporal dementia (FTD), and Pick's Disease. Dementia can also be associated with medical problems such as strokes, brain tumors, brain injuries, and Parkinson's disease, to name a few. All the different forms of dementia, including Alzheimer's, are caused by damaged brain cells (neurons). These damaged neurons disrupt the normal way the brain functions, so that the brain can't do its job. This causes the afflicted person to experience problems in thinking, behavior, emotions and/or movement—and often a combination of all of these. With very few exceptions, dementia is not curable.

COMMON MISCONCEPTIONS ABOUT ALZHEIMER'S AND DEMENTIA

Most people think of Alzheimer's disease only in terms of memory loss. However, the symptoms of Alzheimer's disease also include poor sequencing and planning, poor judgment, *apathy* or loss of initiative, poor insight, trouble with location (getting lost) and confusion.

It is important to realize that the memory disturbance that is the hallmark of Alzheimer's is short-term memory loss. In fact, people are often surprised to realize how much of the distant past a patient with early Alzheimer's can remember. Family members will often comment, "Her memory for the past is great, so I don't think she has Alzheimer's." We like to emphasize to people that short-term memory loss is best understood as the inability to learn **new** material. For example, a patient with Alzheimer's might absolutely believe that his wallet was stolen because he can't remember (or did not learn) that he gave it to his son for safekeeping. No amount of arguing that he never gave his son the wallet will help, because for the patient with Alzheimer's disease, the new information doesn't "stick." This is very important to understand when considering the best ways to interact with people with Alzheimer's.

Another common misconception about Alzheimer's is that of "alertness." We will often hear health care workers confidently assert that a patient does not have Alzheimer's because he is "alert and not confused." Level of alertness describes the extent that someone is awake or aroused—not the degree of confusion or memory loss. In fact, "confusion" is often not apparent in a person with dementia. A person with dementia might appear to be very clear minded and not perplexed at all. However, with careful observation, it will become evident that the person is not in possession of important facts such as day, year, or situation. A problem occurs when we try to identify dementia solely by observing a person's behavior (i.e. "confusion"), rather than examining his or her memory, thinking, and ability to function.

Many people are able to successfully hide their memory and thinking problems for long periods of time because their social skills, such as conversational ability, are still intact. One way to think about this is to remember a time you have been at a party and someone comes up to you and says, "Hi! Do you remember me?" If you don't remember the person, you can still carry on a reasonable conversation for ten or so minutes by "covering" the fact that you don't remember. No one watching would say you were "confused," but the fact remains that you are clueless as to whom you are talking! This is an example of using social skills to cover memory lapse, and many people with Alzheimer's and other dementias can do this long into the progression of their illnesses.

DIAGNOSIS OF DEMENTIA

Lists of dementia warning signs exist, and although it is tempting to look at such a list of symptoms associated with Alzheimer's and try to "diagnose" yourself or a loved one, an accurate diagnosis of Alzheimer's is simply not possible to make without other information. Currently, we make the diagnosis of Alzheimer's disease **clinically**, which just means that we identify a person's symptoms (which almost always requires information from family or friends), make sure the symptoms are not due to other identifiable causes, and then, based on the symptom pattern we see, make a diagnosis. There is not a blood test or brain scan in common use that will reliably differentiate Alzheimer's from other types of dementia. This process of clinical diagnosis sounds simple and straightforward but it is far from easy. As you will see in the discussion below, the symptoms of Alzheimer's disease are similar to those of many other forms of dementia, but can be distinguished by a skilled clinician approximately 90% of the time.

A number of other illnesses can mimic the symptoms of Alzheimer's, and so it's important for a clinician to do the appropriate diagnostic work-up including careful history, physical examination, laboratory, and imaging studies to *rule out* or exclude other treatable causes of the symptoms of dementia. The diagnostic process usually includes a complete medical history, examination, and laboratory testing of blood and urine and brain imaging. The medical history should include questions about family history, psychiatric problems or symptoms, physical complaints, all the medications a person is taking, habits such as alcohol or drug use, and memory symptoms. In order to make sure the medical history is as accurate as possible, a physician may enlist the aid of a family member or spouse.

Neuropsychological testing in which a specialized psychologist will administer an extensive series of mental tests designed to identify and characterize changes in memory, judgment, insight, and planning is sometimes used to help make a diagnosis, but there is no specific neuropsychological test that differentiates Alzheimer's from other dementias. Rather, the identification of Alzheimer's requires an experienced and skilled neuropsychologist who can interpret test results, since many of the abnormalities seen in testing can be due to other causes. The test results are not like taking a test with "right" or "wrong" answers. Instead, the testing reveals patterns of abnormalities. A neuropsychologist must be skilled and experienced in order to interpret the test results properly.

Some physicians, particularly geriatric psychiatrists and certain neurologists, might not routinely use full neuropsychological testing, but regardless of who is doing the examination, any patient with suspected Alzheimer's should undergo a careful clinical examination of thinking known as a *mental status examination.* Sometimes, in the hands of a skilled physician, patients and families might not even notice that the majority of the mental status examination is taking place, because the physician is able to weave the examination questions into conversation. Sometimes physicians are criticized by patients and families who don't understand this. The physician is perceived as "just talking and joking" with the patient. In reality, that "talking and joking" is often the mark of a sophisticated clinician.

ABOUT BRAIN FUNCTION

Now that you have a very basic knowledge of Alzheimer's and other dementias, let's look at how the brain directs behavior. It is very important to remember that the entire brain is interconnected, and communication between the various parts of the brain is crucial. Even if an area if the brain is not damaged, it still might not function properly because **other** areas that communicate with it might be damaged. So, for example, even though the part of your brain that moves your hand might be completely normal, if it doesn't get the signal to turn on and start the hand moving, nothing happens. Just like if you are in a room and someone wants you to turn on the light, but cannot communicate that instruction to you, the light won't come on even though you are capable of turning it on and the electrical circuits are all working fine.

Regrettably, caregivers are often not trained to understand how dementia affects the brain. So, for instance, when a person with Alzheimer's can't follow directions the caregiver will assume that the person is just not motivated or is being disobedient or stubborn. This is akin to always blaming a burned out light bulb when a light won't turn on. Caregivers even get angry at persons with Alzheimer's if the caregiver "explains" and the person still doesn't follow the instructions. You might as well get angry at the light bulb.

Our brain functions can be divided into several general areas: vision, language, memory, executive function, and emotion. Just remember that the brain is interconnected and information is passed from one area to the next and back again. To make this easier, we will go function by function and discuss how the brain operates and how dementia can affect that function.

Vision

When visual information enters the eye, the information travels along the nerve cells through the brain to the back of the brain. Motion, distance, height, length, shading—all this is conveyed through the neurons in the brain and instantaneously received and interpreted. Several areas of the brain work to interpret the visual information and make some sense of it for you by determining angles, depth, texture changes, and spatial relationships. If these areas are damaged, people might not be able to distinguish objects by texture or color or spatial relationships. This is one reason why people with Alzheimer's disease often appear afraid as they cross a threshold into a new room (especially if the room is dark) or are unable to "see" handrails tastefully painted the same color as the wall. In assisted living facilities, the tasteful decorating schemes are more often used to provide a "homey" feel, but if colors and textures are too coordinated, the resident with dementia may not be able to find light switches or handrails that blend in with the decor, or they may not be able to discriminate the closet door from the door to the hallway.

Language

Our brain understands what words mean, and it formulates our thoughts into speech or written words. People with Alzheimer's will pick up a newspaper and focus their attention on the articles and appear to "read." Families will say to us, "He really enjoys his morning newspaper. He reads every section." However, if you ask the person with Alzheimer's to actually read the words or explain the article or headline, he may not be able to do it, because he cannot interpret the information or recognize the words. Sometimes the first sign of dementia can be severely increased problems finding the right words to use when talking, or difficulties coming up with the names of common objects. We all have this problem occasionally, but in Alzheimer's it is to the point that the person has problems communicating with others, and family members are often unable to decipher the message that the affected person is trying to convey. Sometimes the person will use the wrong word for something, resulting in confusion about their message.

The brain also interprets the non-verbal parts of language such as a gesture, a facial expression, or a tone of voice that adds meaning to the words someone says. How do you know when someone is kidding around? If someone smiles or laughs, tilts his head back, and slaps his knee, you might think he has made a joke. If someone is yelling in an angry way at another person, you understand that he is not angry at you, and you most likely keep your distance from the situation.

If your brain has a disease that interferes with its ability to understand verbal and/or non-verbal messages, you might not know whether a person who is yelling is mad at you or calling for help, and you might feel threatened and frightened by them. Teasing and laughing might be misunderstood. A person acting in a hurried manner or using frantic gestures might seem threatening or aggressive.

Memory

Memory is a very complex and misunderstood function of the brain. We know very little about how memories actually get "stored" in our brain cells. We know that emotional reactions, physical conditions like fatigue and illness, and even our own personal biases can affect memory. It is clear that we will often remember things better if we have some emotional association to the information. This is a survival skill, because it allows us to remember things that seem dangerous to us, such as the difference between a friend and an enemy. Many people with Alzheimer's will recall the emotional tone of a situation, even when they don't remember the actual details of the event. That is why it is easier for them to remember if they had a good or bad day, rather than what they actually did all day. This "emotional memory," if you will, is also a reason why they may seem afraid or angry at a particular caregiver. Some event or interaction with that caregiver stirs up a memory, but the person with Alzheimer's cannot express to us the details of the event or conversation.

Earlier we discussed that the memory loss associated with Alzheimer's is short-term memory loss. Practically speaking, this means that someone cannot learn **new** things. Why can a person with memory problems recall where they grew up, or the name of their best friend in high school, but they cannot recall what they had for breakfast, or whether they ate breakfast? Let's use an analogy to help understand how memory loss occurs in Alzheimer's disease. Remember, though, that this is a huge simplification of how memory works and is merely meant to help you conceptualize the process.

Imagine your brain as a file room with rows upon rows of filing cabinets filled with folders which are themselves filled with papers. Information or thoughts come into the room as a piece of paper, and the file clerk must store it. Let's say you want to store the name of the hotel where you will stay at a conference this coming October. "Hmm," your filing clerk says as he looks at the writing and the picture, "Hotel Lamont. That would go in the places stayed section, ...Campsites...Bed & Breakfasts...

Hotels...ah... October meeting...it goes here." He places the paper in the folder, closes the cabinet, and awaits another piece of paper. Later, when someone asks you where you will be staying for your meeting, the file clerk gets the request, goes to the filing cabinet, pulls open the drawer, looks in the folder, and pulls out the paper. "The Hotel Lamont," you say with confidence as you picture the front of the hotel.

Recall that the neurons of someone with Alzheimer's disease are damaged and can't work. In the filing room of someone with Alzheimer's, the papers with new information don't get filed because there are no more folders and filing cabinets available for new information. Sometimes the papers don't even get to the clerk, or by the time they get to the clerk they have the wrong information on them. The papers pile up, sometimes get thrown away entirely, or are lost. The file clerk can retrieve papers from the few existing file cabinets, because the system is already in place. The file clerk can occasionally find a needed paper in the piles of new information which don't have file cabinets, which is always a big thrill, but he cannot always make any sense of the paper he finds. Eventually the clerk quits, so there is no one left even to retrieve papers filed long ago—important papers like how to chew and swallow. So, that is why a person with memory problems can recall where they grew up, or the name of their best friend in high school, but they cannot recall what they had for breakfast, or whether they ate breakfast. The "files" for that old memory were already in place, but the Alzheimer's patient cannot make new "files" for information about today's breakfast.

This is not to say before the filing clerk quits that a person with Alzheimer's cannot learn **anything**. It's just that the learning is typically a very long and difficult process, so it's not reasonable to expect someone with Alzheimer's to learn, "Your daughter will be here in an hour." A person with Alzheimer's can learn routines, as you may have noticed if your loved one in Alzheimer's care knows the times that meals are served. However, part of this is due to the already learned routine of mealtimes over the lifetime.

Such preservation of long-term memories explains why residents with Alzheimer's will try to leave a facility at the end of the day to "pick up the children from school," or to "go home" from work. They will see the staff waving, saying goodbye to each other, and leaving, and a memory is recalled, prompting them to want to "go home." We are sure you have noticed other behaviors that seem to be like the replaying of old scripts, and now you can understand some of the complex memory work that goes into such behaviors.

Executive Function

When other parts of the brain have interpreted what we have seen, heard, smelled, tasted, and touched, they communicate with the frontal lobes, which must decide what to do with all that information and direct the action. Our frontal lobes are the "executive" centers. They put into effect an action plan based on all the information they have received. The frontal lobes are in charge of planning, starting an action, sequencing, logically reasoning, judging, discriminating appropriate actions from inappropriate actions, and stopping a behavior when the goal is reached. Also, the ability to judge the outcome of our actions helps us to learn from our mistakes and to change our behavior as needed.

Another important role of the frontal lobes is to act as the "hand over the mouth," that censors what we say and how we act. This is called *inhibition*. When it fails, it is called *disinhibition*. Alcohol is a very common cause of disinhibition even in people without dementia. Getting tipsy is a very effective way to take the hand away from the mouth and say whatever comes to mind. In other words, the frontal lobes have stopped inhibiting (stopping) someone from engaging in an unacceptable behavior—like dancing around with a lampshade on his head. One distressing behavioral manifestation of disinhibition in dementia is abnormal sexual behavior. Sometimes a person with dementia will say or do sexual things that are completely out of character. This can be very upsetting for families and loved ones. The important thing to remember is this behavior is a result of the disease process and not a moral failing of your loved one.

The frontal lobe functions are the last to develop, and studies report that adolescent frontal lobes are not fully developed. Well, you probably knew that already, but it's good to have some scientific evidence to back up your observations.

Executive dysfunction, rather than memory problems, can be one of the earliest signs of dementia, and in some forms of dementia are characterized almost completely by executive dysfunction. So, the dementia can be missed by others. All too often, we are contacted for help by assisted living facilities because someone is "violent." In reality, that person is simply reacting (without proper frontal lobe function) to a situation. In many cases the environment can be modified rather than using medication to control the behavior. You will read in this book about many similar situations.

Another important and often overlooked function of the frontal lobes is initiation. The initiation component of executive function is what causes us to start an action or activity—the "go button," if you will. Often we see patients with dementia who "won't" come out of their rooms to eat. They might be perfectly aware that it's dinner time, but their go button is missing so they just don't get up to eat. Unless assisted living staff are aware of frontal lobe dysfunction in dementia, they are likely to allow such a resident to skip meals, assuming he or she is not hungry, when, in fact, the resident simply cannot maintain the focus necessary to get to the dining room on his or her own to eat.

Loss of insight is one of the features of impaired executive function. One of the hallmarks of Alzheimer's, and the most distressing to families and friends, is the patient's lack of awareness of any cognitive problems. Families will often say to us that their loved one "just doesn't want to admit" there are problems. The person with dementia knows his or her family is concerned but it is useless to try to convince them that they have deficits and need help, because the frontal lobes are not working as they should, and therefore, the person has absolutely no awareness of his or her problems.

Because the person with Alzheimer's lacks insight into the fact that he has a problem, he may interpret events and others' behaviors in a rather bizarre or paranoid way. After all, if you believe your memory is normal, how do you explain that your wallet is not on your dresser? You **know** you left it there. The only explanation (since you don't realize you have memory problems) is that someone must have stolen it. When the wallet is later found, the person with Alzheimer's may attribute this to the perpetrator's returning the item because of a sudden attack of conscience. This lack of insight is also why it is difficult for families to try to gain control of the finances of the person with dementia. If you believe that you are capable of managing your money and you really intend to take care of those bills, why would you give up your checkbook to a family member? They may spend all your money—after all, they have been stealing your purse.

Hand in hand with loss of insight is a loss of judgment. People retain the ability to give the appropriate answer to hypothetical problems (What would you do if...), but when they are confronted with an actual situation—for example a nice young stranger who asks for money—they will not use appropriate judgment and will give the money away even though they "know" they shouldn't.

SUMMARY

As you can tell by now, basic knowledge of how the brain works is critical to understanding how Alzheimer's affects behavior. At this point in the book, you already know more than most caregivers in facilities that are promoted as providing expert dementia care. Many caregivers, even professional ones, believe that behavior problems are an inevitable part of the disease process and cannot be prevented or resolved. However, as you will find out in this book, one of the main problems is that caregivers have difficulty interpreting behaviors in a way that allows them to develop interventions. They are not trained **why** those behaviors occur or how to determine which brain function is affected. Read on, because when you learn as much as you can about today's long-term care industry, particularly assisted living and specialty dementia care facilities, you can be a better advocate for yourself or a loved one.

CHAPTER TWO
THE DEMENTIA CARE CRISIS

To understand the crisis facing aging Americans, it is important to gain a sense of the enormous scope of Alzheimer's disease and other dementias as well as the associated costs. The information you are about to read is not a secret. Policy makers, health care providers, and legislators know all about this. Ordinary people might not know the actual numbers, but everyone knows someone who has been affected by dementia. So, in a real way, everyone "knows" these numbers, but what do they really mean when you are faced with the diagnosis of dementia in yourself or a loved one? Briefly, these numbers mean that there is a crisis brewing and that if you don't understand the issues, your job in dealing with a new diagnosis of dementia—your own or your loved one's—is much more difficult than it needs to be.

Dementia is an enormous public health problem. There are many kinds of dementia, including Alzheimer's, but the fact is that there is no cure available for any of them in the near future. Currently, about 4.5 million Americans have Alzheimer's disease. One in every three people knows someone with Alzheimer's. Approximately 10% of people in the United States have a family member with the disease. (Ask around and you'll see.) Projections indicate that by the year 2050, the number of people with

Alzheimer's will likely triple to about 16 million. [1] By 2025, six western states will experience at least a 100% increase in the number of residents with Alzheimer's. The three states that already have the largest number of cases are Texas, Florida, and California. By 2025 there will be 74% more cases in Texas, 64% more in Florida, and 50% more in California. [1]

With increasing age, there is increasing risk of developing some form of dementia. The Alzheimer's Association reports that the risk of developing Alzheimer's disease doubles every year after age 65, and by age 85 a person has a 50% chance of having the disease.

The number of young people entering the workforce is not keeping pace with the number of elders leaving the workforce. There will be fewer caregivers available for the increasing elder population with dementia. According to the U.S. Bureau of Labor Statistics, in five years the long-term care industry will need 39% more direct-care staff, but the availability of such staff will rise by only 1.25%, resulting in a drastic shortage of personnel. This is because the "traditional" caregiver is a female between the ages of 25 and 44, and the population in this age group is not growing but has reached a plateau, while the population needing care—namely the elderly—is increasing. [2]

Our current health care entitlements for the elderly (Medicare and, to some extent, Medicaid) will be insufficient to cover the cost of care for the ballooning dementia population. The cost of medical care will rise exponentially. In the year 2010, Medicare will spend 54.5% more for Alzheimer's health care, and Medicaid-reimbursed costs for residential (i.e., nursing home and Medicaid-waiver residences) care will rise 80%. Care costs in general are 200% more for those in later, more severe stages of the disease than those for those in the earlier stages. In and of themselves, those figures are staggering, but they are even more worrisome when you consider that the estimates are for Alzheimer's disease alone, which is only one of many different types of dementia, all of which ultimately result in difficulties with daily functioning to the point that people usually need additional care.

Better care will not mean more care. It will mean smarter care, and this is not happening now. Increasing the "warehousing" facilities for those with dementia will not solve the crisis. What is necessary is that families understand dementia so that they can demand proper care. Caregivers must understand the disease so that they can provide the care that families demand and elders deserve.

All the statistics above are alarming, but what is most worrisome is the fact that staff caregivers in assisted living facilities have limited knowledge and training about dementia and the behaviors associated with such brain disorders. The Alzheimer's Association cites studies that indicate at least two-thirds of all assisted living residents have some mental health problem, and half of the residents have dementia. [3] In 2000, assisted living facilities were studied by the U.S. Department of Health and Human Services (DHHS), which noted that direct-care staff in assisted living facilities were knowledgeable about patient care, such as "physical health problems," and "medication management, with the exception of antipsychotic medications," but "had no clear picture of normal aging." [4] We provide more information about this aspect of the crisis in other chapters of this book.

These statistics and trends boil down to very real dilemmas for individual elders and their families.

Clearly, many people have recognized these realities and are working hard to rectify the situation. In the meantime, what alternatives do families have for weathering the coming elder-care storm? First, let's look at the general kinds of options available.

THE CURRENT LANDSCAPE: COMMONLY AVAILABLE CARE OPTIONS

In the past, families needing to assist elderly loved ones had few options besides taking care of them in their homes. They could also hire private caregivers or could "place" their family member in a nursing home. Neither option was optimum, since private caregivers were expensive, untrained and often unreliable, and nursing homes had come to symbolize "the end of the road" warehousing of the elderly. Now there are more choices for families, so let's look at some of the general options available.

Adult Day Care (Senior Day Programs)

Adult day care has evolved to give daily respite to caregivers of those living at home with dementia. These are particular care centers with specialized programs, caregivers, and even architecture catering to the needs of those with Alzheimer's and other dementias. This type of care provides social contact, supervised activity, meals, and, in many cases, routine medication administration. Many of these centers have transportation services, which can further increase the convenience for families. Medicare does not pay for adult day care, although in some states and for some programs, Medicaid will pay. Adult day care may be covered by long-term care insurance, depending on the type of coverage one has. However, adult day care might or might not be sufficient for home care of an elderly person with dementia.

Non-medical Home Care

Essentially, non-medical home care, which is also referred to as custodial care or companion care, offers services including housekeeping, bathing, dressing, cooking, driving, activities, and shopping. Large companies now provide registered, "trained," and bonded caregivers and offer some reassurance that the in-home caregiver will be more reliable and educated about the needs of an elder with dementia. Some families choose to find in-home caregivers through an agency, and other families choose to find their own "freelance" caregiver(s). Although caregivers retained through an agency are often more expensive than those who are not, there are some advantages to hiring a caregiver through a reputable agency. First, if the caregiver doesn't show up, an agency will typically stand behind their pledge to furnish help in the home. In other words, you have recourse if a caregiver is absent or tardy. Second, the caregivers theoretically have some professional oversight by the managers of the company, and you are less likely to have someone in your home who has legal or other problems.

Medicare pays for home health care, but there are significant restrictions on the types and duration of care provided. So-called custodial care, or companion care, is not paid for by Medicare, although it might be covered by some long-term care insurance policies.

Assisted Living

Assisted living facilities, including small homes, were established as a better option for providing services to older people who did not need skilled nursing care in a nursing home but whose needs were more intensive than could be provided at home—either for reasons of actual caregiving or for social contact unavailable at home. The idea behind assisted living was to provide a place where elders could maintain a level of independence but have security and help available whenever needed. These new facilities were more "home-like" and, unlike nursing homes, sought to avoid any resemblance to hospitals. Families could relax because mom or dad would be in a pleasant place with meals, activities, social events, transportation, and nursing assistance. Assisted living became a welcome relief to many families and elders needing help. Medicare does not pay for any part of assisted living. In some states, Medicaid will pay for assisted living.

The National Center for Assisted Living (NCAL) estimates there are 33,000 assisted living facilities in the United States. The number of people in assisted living communities is estimated to be about 1 million. More than 75% of residents are female and the rest are male. [5] According to the Assisted Living Federation of America (ALFA), the number of facilities owned, leased, and managed by the largest 50 U.S. assisted living companies in 2007 was about 2700. The top 10 companies provide space for about 110,000 residents. [6]

Nursing Homes

Mrs. Jackson: "Lady of Leisure"

Tiny Mrs. Jackson lived in a nursing home because she was in the later stages of Alzheimer's. She was a nice lady except when it came time for her shower. Every morning, during the nursing home's standard shower time, Mrs. Jackson would yell and hit the staff when they came to wake her for her shower. Lately she had become more aggressive and would actually bite staff as they tried to take off her pajamas. In the shower, she would scream and yell and would use her fists to fight the aides. The staff caregivers were at their wits' end, so the social worker called Mrs. Jackson's daughter, who lived in another city, to tell her that the staff could not handle Mrs. Jackson's behavior. Mrs. Jackson's daughter was understandably confused by her usually sweet mother's inexplicable aggression, but the social worker reassured her that physical aggression is common in people with dementia and, for some, an inevitable part of the disease. Mrs. Jackson's daughter had never known her mother to be aggressive, but she had not visited in a few weeks, so she trusted the reports of the staff. The social worker explained that the policy of the facility in cases of aggression was to call the resident's doctor to request a prescription for medication to calm the individual. She told Mrs. Jackson's daughter that the nursing staff had already done this, and Mrs. Jackson was now doing "fine."

Mrs. Jackson's daughter immediately made plane reservations to visit her mother, but after her arrival, she found her mother sleeping every time she visited. After a week of this, she went to the administrator of the facility and complained. The nursing supervisor said there was no other way to manage Mrs. Jackson's behavior except by using medication because she was injuring the staff, and they were becoming afraid to take care of her. Besides, she said, they had a routine schedule, and dealing with Mrs. Jackson's behavior was making aides late to care for other residents.

Mrs. Jackson's daughter refused to accept these explanations and began to ask questions. The aides said that every day when they woke her mother up at 6:30 AM, she would bite them and yell. Mrs. Jackson's daughter was stunned because she had taken great care during the admission process to explain to both the social worker and the director of nursing that Mrs. Jackson never awakened before 10 AM. In fact, it was a joke in the family that Mrs. Jackson was a "lady of leisure" because she liked to sleep late in the morning. Mrs. Jackson's daughter had also emphasized that her mother always took her shower in the evening before going to bed because it relaxed her. After learning of the facility's failure to accommodate the habits of her mother, Mrs. Jackson's daughter requested that the doctor take her mother off the medicines and that the staff try a different schedule for bathing and dressing. The nurse reluctantly agreed to call the doctor and make the request and instructed the staff not to go into Mrs. Jackson's room the next morning until 10 AM.

When an aide came in the following morning, Mrs. Jackson was sleeping. The aide gently touched her shoulder and called her name, then moved away from the bed, expecting to be yelled at. Instead, Mrs. Jackson opened her eyes and gave the aide a slight smile. The aide told her that today she would be showered before bedtime. At shower time, Mrs. Jackson complained that the water was "too hot," but when proper temperature adjustments were made, she relaxed, as did the aide. Mrs. Jackson's daughter was relieved that her mother would be able to continue to be cared for at the same facility—but in the future with respect and dignity—and the staff was glad that they could so easily make Mrs. Jackson's day and their own more pleasant.

Many families of residents in nursing homes have experienced situations similar to that of Mrs. Jackson. Because of the institutional regimentation, little consideration is given to the residents' individual and unique needs. These common experiences of families have resulted in unpleasant stereotypes and enduring media images of residents in wheelchairs lined up in the hallway. For this reason assisted living arose as an alternative to what is considered institutional care.

If you try to find an actual definition for nursing home, you will see that there is little in the definition that will differentiate a nursing home from assisted living. Both provide 24-hour care for residents needing assistance with activities of daily living. Overall, the biggest practical distinction between nursing homes and assisted living facilities lies in their philosophies about caring for their residents. Nursing homes were and usually still are modeled on a medical model of care. You will often see rooms that look like hospital rooms, usually in a roommate set-up. A patient's physician will visit the nursing home on a regular basis. There is nursing care given in nursing homes, and usually a nursing station. The residents of nursing homes are typically more physically debilitated than those of assisted living, and many are bedridden. The rate of dementia in nursing homes is high, but there are also patients who are in nursing homes largely because of physical needs. Within the last 15 years, a specialized niche has developed for nursing homes to act as short-term rehabilitation centers covered by Medicare. Patients who have had recent hospitalization may be discharged to nursing homes as a step-down option for rehabilitation services (including occupational therapy, physical therapy, and speech therapy) paid for by Medicare.

Regardless of the medical model, nursing homes are not bound to impersonal care. As we saw with Mrs. Jackson, small changes can make a big difference in the quality of a resident's life.

Specialty Dementia Care Facilities

Specialized dementia care facilities are considered a form of assisted living in that they are not based on a medical model, do not provide acute rehabilitation services, and are not typically covered by public entitlement programs such as Medicare or Medicaid. However, some long-term care insurance policies will pay for the care. These specialized dementia facilities are sometimes housed in a dedicated wing or unit within a facility (either nursing home or assisted living), or they might be free-standing yet affiliated with facilities providing other levels of care. In some cases they might be completely independent. They are typically secured, meaning the doors are locked to prevent residents from wandering out into the street or neighborhood. The locked front door can seem forebidding at first, but the safety of the confines of the facility can be quite reassuring for those families whose loved one has been found in the middle of the night in a neighbor's front yard or become lost in the grocery store parking lot. Most of these specialized dementia care centers are not always required to provide additional staffing and programming to assist residents with dementia. As you will see in the next story, even residents with dementia can have medical emergencies or problems.

Kelly's Mother's Disastrous Yet "Unavoidable" Fall

Kelly had just finished a business meeting and was on her way to pick up her sick daughter from school when she received a telephone call. "Kelly, this is Belinda, the social worker from your mother's assisted living. I am sorry to tell you that your mother had an accident and was sent to the emergency room." Kelly's thoughts immediately raced to try to catch up with the frightening news. She had reluctantly placed her mother, Eunice, in the Alzheimer's care facility only last month, expecting that the staff would give her mother the specialized care needed for her condition. As she worried about her mother, Kelly also thought through all of the obligations she had that day; she was able to contact her husband to pick up her daughter and fortunately, Kelly's supervisor was generous and would allow her an extra day to send in the report on that day's business meeting, but the company was talking about layoffs. . . . She couldn't think about that now. She had to concentrate on her mother.

Upon arriving at the emergency room, Kelly found her mother unresponsive. There was a harried ER doctor who quickly began asking Kelly for information about the fall. Kelly was confused. "Do you mean that the assisted living didn't send someone here with Mother?" she asked. Hearing the negative reply, Kelly's confidence in the heart-wrenching decision she had made to put her mother in assisted living was badly shaken. This was to be the first of many unpleasant realizations on Kelly's journey into the real world of dementia care.

In trying to assist the emergency room staff with obtaining medical information necessary to treat her mother, Kelly gleaned disturbing insights into what had happened at the assisted living earlier that day. She discovered that her mother had been sitting unsupervised in the day area with eight other residents, some of them prone to the violent outbursts that may be part of Alzheimer's disease as it progresses. A staff member (one of two nursing assistants responsible for the majority of the 36 residents' day-to-day care) had attempted to wake a particularly aggressive male resident as he was dozing by shaking his shoulders from behind while loudly calling "Hey, Lazybones, get up!" The male resident, a WWII combat veteran, awoke startled, and yelled in fear while he attempted to attack the nursing assistant. When Kelly's mother, who was confused and upset by the angry confrontation, tried to intervene, the male resident knocked her into the sharp corner of a marble-top table in the area.

Kelly learned that her mother had sustained massive brain hemorrhaging as a result of the incident. She also found that after the accident had occurred, her mother had not been evaluated by the LVN on duty for over 30 minutes because none of the professional staff at the assisted living facility had recognized that her increased confusion and the sudden onset of poor muscle coordination might be signs of a more serious problem. The staff became concerned only after Eunice was unable to eat her snack unaided. Even at that point, only her vital signs had been recorded. When she had a seizure, the staff had called for the ambulance and sent her to the local emergency room for evaluation.

Kelly tried to understand how this could happen to her mother in one of the best Alzheimer's facilities in the city. She talked to Belinda, the social worker, but was informed that she was a part-time employee who only helped residents complete forms for government benefits. The social worker admitted to Kelly that although she had urged the administration to provide specialized behavioral training for the assisted living staff, the corporation that owned the facility provided training only one day a year for the entire staff. Besides, the administration was confident that the training required by the state regulatory agencies was adequate.

Thinking that the assisted living workers had been trained properly but that somehow their training had failed to help them prevent her mother's injury, Kelly thought she might learn more if she spoke with the facility's director, Susan, who was not a nurse, but an administrator/manager. Apparently, the facility was not required by the state to have a qualified registered nurse or a licensed vocational nurse on staff. Susan told Kelly, "These things just happen, and your mother should have known better than to try to help out in a fight. I'm sure the other resident didn't intend to hurt her, but he's always mean to other people, anyway. You really cannot control some demented patients without large doses of medication or restraints, and, of course, we are a patient-centered and restraint-free community." Because Kelly had believed that this particular assisted living home was the premier dementia care facility in the community, she was stunned by Susan's attitude and ignorance about behavioral disturbances associated with dementia.

It is not surprising that the professional staff at the assisted living facility did not recognize Kelly's mother's brain injury, given their mistaken belief that significant changes in a resident's behavior are simply part of the progression of Alzheimer's disease and not due to a medical problem.

PROBLEMS WITH ASSISTED LIVING

As you have probably already surmised, one thing that all of the above care models have in common is a woeful inadequacy in training of caregiver staff. In our opinion, this inadequate training is probably the prime factor in the growing crisis in long-term care for people with

Alzheimer's disease and other forms of dementia. We have limited the scope of this book to assisted living, but the care issues discussed could be applied to adult day care, non-medical home care, and specialized dementia care homes or facilities.

Definition of Assisted Living

The National Center for Assisted Living (NCAL) states that there is an "absence of a common definition for assisted living." [8] In one way, the diffuse nature of assisted living is useful in that it provides more options to elders seeking assisted living, although the wide diversity can lead to the lack of a standard for quality of care, staffing, or services, but in our opinion, the problems seen in assisted living are greatly exacerbated by its lack of cohesive identity.

Depending on the state where one lives, assisted living may be called board-and-care, residential care, or personal care home, for instance. Assisted living can be any size—from a small home with three or four residents to a large multi-story structure with hundreds of residents. Assisted living can mean one's own efficiency-type apartment, a bedroom with a bath, a bedroom with shared bathroom, or even a shared bedroom and bath. The good thing about the diffuse nature of assisted living is that there are lots of options available to elders seeking assisted living; at the same time, the wide diversity can mean lack of standards for quality of care, staffing, or services.

The wide variety of definitions and regulations of assisted living dementia care from state to state makes it even more difficult for families to seek out the best care for loved ones with Alzheimer's disease. Suppose Mr. Smith's daughter in Iowa looks for a facility to place her father near his current home in Orlando, Florida. It would be comforting and more efficient if she knows that assisted living is similarly defined and monitored in Florida as in Iowa. Given our mobile culture and the long distance relationships in families, there is a demand for sameness, or at least comparability. Caregiver training requirements (if they are in place) also vary widely from state to state. For instance, Mr. Smith's daughter can call a plumber in Florida to fix her father's toilet and be assured that the plumber's knowledge is comparable to her plumber in Iowa. However, that is not true of caregiver expertise from state to state.

Of course, plumbing cannot be directly compared to the care of frail elderly, but consumers need and want the ability to compare services and skills. The issue of caregiver training requirements leads us to what we believe is one of the most serious problem in assisted living: lack of regulatory oversight.

In our experience, families are attracted to assisted living because of the "homelike" atmosphere and level of independence they afford the residents. Consumers see assisted living as a place where it is reasonable to expect seniors to live without being "institutionalized." People move into assisted living with a vague expectation of having to move to a higher level of care in the future, and the recently popularized trend of "aging in place" aims to provide the longest care possible at a single facility. Elders currently residing in assisted living are purportedly better off than those persons in a nursing home or living alone without help. However, one cannot paint a positive picture of assisted living with a broad stroke. There are a number of problems that make choosing a facility very difficulty, and, at times, risky.

Lack of Regulatory Oversight

What most people also do not know is that assisted living, adult day care, and non-medical home care have not received the same regulatory scrutiny as nursing homes, which have come under strict federal and state control since the well-known investigations of substandard care that resulted in federal regulation in 1987. According to the Consumer Consortium of Assisted Living (CCAL), "There are no federal regulations or uniform standards of operation for assisted living. Each state develops their assisted living regulations separately and differently. Some states began forming assisted living regulation as facilities began operation in their state. Other states lagged in this effort and only began addressing regulation in the past several years." [9] Until very recently, some states, such as Pennsylvania, had no regulations over assisted living.

While people's initial reaction to learning that there are no federal regulations for assisted living is one of dismay, it is important to remember that regulations cannot improve care, because the care is not what is regulated. The process of care—that is, the procedures and the documentation—is regulated.

Federal regulatory controls work by penalizing facilities for things that go wrong—based on mathematical formulas and data sets. So the focus of abiding by regulations becomes one of avoidance of punishment for things that may have little to do with quality care. Inevitably, when systems strive to conform to a minimally expected norm, excellence is discouraged because the very attempt to reach excellence requires a certain amount of daring—of reaching beyond the norm. If only the norm is measured by those in authority, then people are not willing to risk missing the norm while attempting the excellent. In other words, the lowest common denominator is rewarded.

The intent of the public's desire for regulation is to institute meaningful and positive changes in the way facilities take care of residents. However, as seen in the nursing home industry, the avoidance of punishment overshadows the real care issues. Before repeating the process that regulated nursing homes 20 years ago, consumers must consider how regulations will change assisted living for the better and for the worse. In other words, be careful what you ask for.

Cost

As stated earlier, Medicare does not pay for any assisted living or private caregiver services that are provided in an assisted living community. In 2006 the cost of a private assisted living residence unit averaged about $2,627 per month per resident, based on a recent survey of facilities. [10] The range of cost is about $1,000 to $4,400 per year, depending on the area of the country. [11] These numbers are for residents requiring little specialized care. The cost of specialized dementia care can be two to three times those amounts. In cases that require extra-close care, or when families want the reassurance of continual caregivers present with their loved one, the cost of a private caregiver is additional to the cost of the assisted living facility. As you can see, the prices of assisted living care are out of reach for many elders and their families. Again, though, in the quest for government entitlement programs to cover the cost of assisted living, consumers should beware. If the cost of care is covered by federal programs such as Medicare, federal regulation inevitably follows. Funding can be withheld for "noncompliance" with federal regulations or mandates. Also, as has previously been the case with Medicare, when federal budgetary constraints occur, Medicare and Medicaid benefits often are the first to be cut.

CAREGIVER DEFICIENCIES

If you can locate an assisted living community, afford the cost, and accept that the facility may not have optimal oversight of its operations, you still must face caregiver deficiencies. Besides the serious deficiencies in caregiver training (see Chapter 3), there are problems with caregiver supply, knowledge, and responsiveness. There is also the risk of abuse of elders who reside in the facility.

Number of Staff

The number of people available and willing to work as caregivers is not keeping up with the number of people who need care. Shortages in nursing staff in hospitals are a major concern, but there are also nursing shortages, as well as shortages of nurses' aides, in long-term care facilities. Recall from earlier in this chapter that U.S. Census information reveals the availability of caregivers lags far behind the booming aging population. This will only worsen over the next 30 years.

There is much debate about how many nurses and aides are needed to care for residents in long-term care. The question is "What is the adequate staff-to-resident ratio, as it is termed, in order to provide quality care?" Some profess that the ratio is not a major contributor to quality of care, but it all depends on how one defines quality of care. Some profess that standards cannot be established, because the needs of residents vary from facility to facility. Regardless, our experience has been that a major complaint made by families and residents in long-term care is the understaffing of the facility.

Knowledge of Staff

About one-third of residents in facilities (including assisted living) surveyed in one study have "moderate to severe cognitive impairment."[3] This is a real problem, because 88% of the staff in the survey by the U.S. Department of Health and Human Services thought that incontinence, memory loss, and confusion are part of normal aging; 78% believed that depression is normal for the elderly; and 63% believed frequent outbursts of anger were a normal part of the aging process. Twenty-one percent (21%) reported that they had no idea of the potentially treatable behaviors or symptoms that should be reported to a nurse or the physician. [4] This means that most of the staff in assisted living facilities would not report behaviors or changes in behavior that could be treated, such as lack of appetite, sudden confusion, or even depression, thus jeopardizing the care provided for the residents.

However, one cannot blame the workers entirely for their lack of knowledge. In 2003 the Seattle Times reported that assisted living providers were trying to overturn state rules that would require them to provide more training for employees and more nursing staff to monitor the residents' medical needs. The reason? The corporations operating the facilities say it would cost too much and warn that the costs would then be passed on to consumers. [7] Chapter 3 details the deficiencies in caregiver training and the poor response by the assisted living industry.

Responsiveness of Staff

There is another disturbing result of the lack of caregivers' knowledge. Often, assisted living staff, including those in management, tell the family that disruptive behaviors are inevitable in the progression of their loved one's disease and that there is little to do but to use tranquilizing medications to control the behavior. Frequently, the family also is told that there are not enough staff caregivers to provide high levels of attention to residents and they are given the "option" of hiring privately paid caregivers to provide the extra help the facility cannot. Of course, the unspoken message to family is that without either medication or private caregivers, the resident can no longer stay in the facility.

The following story is an egregious situation that exemplifies the result of caregiver deficiencies, even after sincere promises were made:

Mrs. O'Neill's Bad Night

Ninety-two-year-old Mrs. O'Neill had recently been moved from the nursing unit of an eldercare facility, where she had been receiving physical therapy following fracture of her femur, to its assisted living unit. Mrs. O'Neill's daughter had been assured her mother would receive the highest level of care, including bathroom assistance and nighttime checks by aides at 2-hour intervals through the night until she adjusted to her new environment. On a Friday two weeks after her move to assisted living, the call device above her bed ceased working. Her daughter, who was very concerned about the problem, was told the maintenance staff could not fix it until the following Monday but not to worry because the aides on evening duty would be checking on her mother every 2 hours. Her daughter was not pleased with this response but decided to "let it lie" until Monday and then take it up with the nursing supervisor first thing on Monday.

The next morning, Mrs. O'Neill called her daughter to report that although there had been regular, 2-hour checks on her the first part of the night, no one had checked on her after midnight. She had awakened in the early morning hours, having urinated in her bed while asleep, and had been afraid to get out of bed to go to the bathroom without assistance. With no way to call for assistance, she had lain awake in her own urine for hours, waiting for an aide to check on her and help her to the bathroom to clean up. When no one appeared, Mrs. O'Neill decided to use her walker to get through the door of her room into the hallway, which she managed to do but with great effort. Once in the hallway, she saw no one so had waited for half an hour next to the aide's station for an aide to appear. Still no one! Eventually she had given up and managed to get back in her room, again with great effort, and had done her best to clean herself in her bathroom. Distraught and frustrated, Mrs. O'Neill had not slept the rest of the evening. No aide came to her room to check on her until approximately 5:30 that morning.

In this story, Mrs. O'Neill did not have dementia, and she was able to at least attempt to take care of her situation and seek help. Imagine the outcome if she had Alzheimer's. Perhaps she might have screamed or called out for help repeatedly, only to be identified by staff as "agitated" and requiring medications. Perhaps her daughter would have been told that the staff cannot be available all the time, and that she needed to hire an extra caregiver for the evenings. You can understand how a simple thing as a broken call button can wreak havoc when staff do not anticipate problems and make appropriate alternative plans for care.

ELDER ABUSE

Although overmedication, poor care, and expulsion from facilities are bad enough, perhaps the most chilling potential problem that exists in some elder care facilities is reflected in the harrowing tales of elder abuse or neglect that have been detailed in the media. In May 2004, both the *Washington Post* and *USA Today* published series of articles about problems in assisted living. The stories reported included rape, inadequate staffing, poor training, medication errors, and acceptance of residents who were too ill and could not receive appropriate care. The response from the assisted living industry typically calls these instances of abuse isolated events or implies that some residents may have been placed in the wrong type of care or that families who are dissatisfied with care can just move their loved ones to a better facility.

When we have tried to discuss the media coverage of these kinds of neglect with some of our friends and colleagues who work for large corporations that own numerous assisted living communities, they have seemed unimpressed with the stories, believing that it could never happen in their particular facilities. Some people have dismissed our concerns by countering that "things are always going to happen." The general opinion seems to be that, because of the nature of dementia, there was very little control over residents' behaviors that could have been exercised in the incidents of abuse and neglect reported in the media. These people usually have followed up with comments regarding the high quality of training that staff caregivers receive at their particular facility and the process of selecting residents who would not be a problem.

THE BIG PICTURE

So now you know there is an increasing number of people with Alzheimer's disease and other forms of dementia, fewer people to take care of them, increased burden on Medicare and Medicaid for coverage of long-term care costs, and a system of long-term care that is out of the financial reach of most people. These factors are indeed critical, but we believe that the more frightening aspects of the crisis are the abysmal level of caregivers' knowledge and the highly variable commitment among administrators to increase caregivers' knowledge and training, even among facilities owned by the same corporation.

If you are not convinced, consider the following situation. What if you went to the day-care center to pick up your 3-year-old son and found him in the parking lot, wandering between cars? What if the day-care supervisor told you that the center just doesn't have enough staff to watch each child every minute? What if the supervisor told you that all the staff was needed in the activity area at that time of day? Also, what if you were told that they would have a long talk with your 3-year-old about safety issues and the necessity of following the schedule to come in at a certain time? What if they suggested you hire your own personal day-care provider to be with your child at the center each day as a solution to his "wandering" behavior? What if they asked you to sign a waiver that you acknowledge your son wanders and that you promise not to hold the day-care center liable if he wanders away and gets hurt? Would you walk away thinking, "Oh well, they're right. Wandering around is just part of what 3-year-old kids do. It's too stressful to find another day-care center. Besides, all the other day-care facilities are the same." Of course not! But this is analogous to what happens daily to families whose loved ones are in assisted living and dementia care units, and, amazingly, families have put up with it.

Use of this example is not to say that an elderly resident in a long-term care facility should be treated like a child and not afforded the same dignity and respect shown any adult. However, the brain of a person with Alzheimer's or another form of dementia cannot process information, make plans, or sequence activities. Staff caregivers have to assist with—and even take over—these functions for a person with dementia. Even if there is limited staff, they are supposed to be trained to determine a way to prevent accidents and keep residents safe.

So then, must families accept a quality of care lower than what they expect for themselves or their children? No, and families are becoming increasingly frustrated by the system of care that has evolved. The assisted living industry has tried to make changes, but so far, very few of the changes that have been instituted seem to be working. The industry continues to grow and increase its wealth, but families continue to feel disenfranchised and their loved ones continue to receive inadequate care, sometimes putting them at risk to the point of outright neglect or even abuse. Families and residents in facilities do not need to feel helpless or just accept that optimal care is not possible. All consumers—families and residents—need more information about aging, dementia, behaviors associated with dementia, and the appropriate ways to manage the behaviors. If you read this book in its entirety, you will know more than the majority of caregivers, managers, and supervisors working in assisted living. Get ready and read on.

REFERENCES

1. Alzheimer's Association. 2008 Alzheimer's Disease Facts and Figures. Available at: http://alz.org/national/documents/report_alzfactsfigures2008.pdf; accessed July 17, 2008.

2. Dawson, Stephen L. Long-Term Care Financing and the Long-Term Care Workforce Crisis: Causes and Solutions. (Prepared for the Citizens for Long-term Care.) Bronx, NY: Paraprofessional Healthcare Institute, January 2003.

3. Gruber-Baldini, Ann L, Boustani, Malaz, Sloane, Philip D, and Zimmerman, Sheryl. Behavioral symptoms in residential care/assisted living facilities: prevalence, risk factors, and medication management. *Journal of the American Geriatrics Society* 2004:52(10);1610-1617.

4. Hawes, Catherine, and Phillips, Charles D. High Service or High Privacy Assisted Living Facilities, Their Residents and Staff: Results from a National Survey. Washington, DC: U.S. Department of Health and Human Services, November 2000.

5. The National Center for Assisted Living Assisted living resident profile. Available at: www.ncal.org/about/resident.cfm; accessed July 17, 2008.

6. Assisted Living Federation of America. 2007 Largest providers. Available at: www.alfa.org/i4a/pages/Index.cfm?pageID=4143; accessed July 17, 2008.

7. King, Marsha. Providers fighting assisted-living rules that would raise standards. *Seattle Times* September 8, 2003.

8. The National Center for Assisted Living. Consumer information. Available at: www.ncal.org/consumer/index.cfm; accessed July 17, 2008.

9. Consumer Consortium on Assisted Living. Frequently asked questions: How is assisted living regulated? Available at: www.ccal.org; accessed December 23, 2004.

10. The National Center for Assisted Living. Assisted living facility profile. Available at: www.ncal.org/about/facility.cfm; accessed July 17, 2008.

11. Eldercare Locator. Fact sheets. Available at: www.eldercare.gov/eldercare/Public/resources/fact_sheets/assisted_living.asp; accessed July 17, 2008.

CHAPTER THREE
THE SORRY STATE OF CAREGIVER TRAINING

Bob and Mary

Bob, who had Alzheimer's disease, had been taken care of at home by his wife, Mary, for the past several years. When they were younger and had planned for their long-term health care needs, they had invested in a long-term care insurance policy. It would pay for either a day-care program or a home caregiver, but not both. Neither had realized at the time that the choice of coverage for either a home caregiver or a day-care program was completely inadequate for the needs of someone with Alzheimer's. Because Mary was on a limited income and wanted to care for Bob herself, she decided that her best option was day care.

Mary's only respite from taking care of Bob was during the several hours each day that Bob would spend at a seniors' day-care program. There, he enjoyed playing board games, listening to music, interacting with other people, eating lunch, and looking at the newspaper. During the time Bob was away, Mary could exercise, run errands, or take a nap. However, she had to be sure to be home when the day-care transportation service dropped Bob off at 3 PM. This was because once he left day care, Bob could not be left alone and Mary had no one to assist her.

Mary had not slept through the night for years because Bob would repeatedly get up to go to the toilet. Usually he would not get there in time, and Mary would have to clean him up before putting him back to bed. On one occasion he became confused and tried to get into the bathroom by pushing against a window. The windowpane broke, seriously cutting his hands and arms. In addition, Bob often fell or knocked over furniture as he tried to get up in the night to leave or start to get dressed, all in a state of confusion. He had stopped talking and had difficulty letting other people know what he wanted or needed. Because his physical weakness and repeated injuries were becoming increasingly hard for her to manage, and because she was so emotionally exhausted, Mary reluctantly decided to place Bob in a dementia care assisted living facility where he would be safe and round-the-clock help would be available. She looked at a number of different facilities and finally chose one that had a reputation for providing the best dementia care in town. To pay the cost of approximately $3,500 per month, Mary would have to use her own pension to fund Bob's care.

Mary cried almost continuously for days after Bob's move to the assisted living facility, not only because she missed him but also because she felt that she had failed him. Mary also worried that Bob would be upset in a strange environment. She was also concerned by the wide variation in age and experience among the caregivers at the facility. Fortunately, though, Bob seemed calm in his new environment and cooperated with the people who took care of him. Besides, the administrator and the staff had assured her that Bob would receive whatever care he needed, at any time of the day.

Mary was actively involved in Bob's care, and she

visited him at length every day. She began to notice, however, that Bob was not eating well. The aides would merely place his tray in front of him and expect him to feed himself. Mary knew that when he had been at home, Bob would often simply sit and look at the food. Because of the changes in his brain from the Alzheimer's disease, he literally could not pick up the fork and start to eat unless someone helped him. Even then, he would take inordinately large bites of food and not stop to swallow. At home, Mary had used a baby's spoon to control the size of his bites, but even then, she only gave him half a spoonful. Because she knew of Bob's difficulty eating, she made sure to talk to the assisted living facility's director of nursing about assisting him during mealtime. Evidently, this message was not conveyed to the other staff caregivers. Besides, there were always so many new caregivers replacing the ones who quit, it was hard for Mary to keep up with who knew anything about her husband.

The problem became even more serious. One day, when lunch was over, the aide came over to Bob and began to remove his tray of food. Bob had not eaten very much of his meal and he reached out and held the aide's arm. The young aide did not understand Bob's behavior; she was startled and, without saying anything, grabbed his arm and tried to remove it from her own. Instinctively, Bob held on tighter. The aide roughly pulled her arm from Bob's grasp, but he continued to reach for her as she took his tray away.

After this incident, the aide reported him as being agitated and aggressive. The director of nursing called Mary and told her that they were going to have to call the doctor for some medication to reduce Bob's aggressive behavior toward the staff. Mary questioned her in some detail, finding out that this was the only episode of agitation.

Mary was told by the nurse that the facility could not provide Bob with individual attention at mealtime because they had to take care of other residents. Besides, she was told, if Bob could not eat on his own, they would just have to move him to a nursing home. Mary struck a deal with the nurse, telling her that she would come at every meal to assist feeding Bob. Mary reasoned that then Bob would not have to be put on medications that she believed would probably only make him sleepy and less functional. She also would not have to put herself and Bob in more distress by moving him to another facility. Mary assumed that she had to be satisfied with what she got, because the facility where Bob lived was reportedly the best one in town. She went to the facility three or more times every day until he died months later.

Unfortunately, as illustrated in Bob's story, staff members were not familiar with Bob's condition and the ways that Alzheimer's disease and other forms of dementia can affect a life function as fundamental as eating. Reduced initiative, inability to complete a sequence of actions, and even swallowing problems can cause eating difficulties. In the above example, the staff member was not trained to approach Bob in ways that would make him feel at ease. She did not understand that, because his communication was limited, he would use gestures or movements to convey a message. She also did not understand that people with dementia cannot interpret others' behaviors and may feel threatened when touched brusquely or when spoken to loudly. Rather than determine the conditions that elicited the "agitation," staff assumed that his behavior was simply a sign of his dementia and that the only means of managing the "agitated" behavior was medication. Analyzing the situation and creating a behavior-management plan would have been much easier and more effective if the staff had been aware of how Bob's brain disease affected him. If the staff had been taught how dementia affects the brain and how to anticipate behavior problems rather than merely react to them, this situation likely would not have occurred. However, this level of staff training and knowledge is usually not the case, which is precisely the problem with the current state of dementia care.

This scenario does not represent an isolated incident but rather one that occurs with disturbing frequency every day across the country. Every day, people receive diagnoses of dementia, and every day, their families struggle to find ways to care for those they love. Information on Alzheimer's and dementia abounds, but caregivers are hindered by lack of time, and difficulty finding a central source of expert advice. Most families, unfortunately, learn "on the job" how to care for a loved one with dementia. We have been told countless times by exhausted caregivers after months and sometimes years of doing their best that they would have paid "anything" to have had our advice from the outset. With this book we hope to give you access to our combined experience in helping people with all aspects of their dementia so that you can be well-equipped from the beginning and avoid the panic and frustration that cripples many people as they face a diagnosis of dementia.

WHAT TRAINING?

If you are surprised by the lack of knowledge of the caregivers in the above example, which describes a specialized Alzheimer's, or dementia care facility, you will be shocked to learn just how little knowledge there is in assisted living communities that are **not** specifically designed to care for residents with dementia. Most of the training provided to employees who work in assisted living facilities focuses on emergency procedures, resident's rights, safety, and fire evacuation. While this training imparts skills that are certainly important and can save lives, the behaviors of a person with Alzheimer's disease or another type of dementia create significant additional risks, requiring specialized training above and beyond the basic requirements. Remember from Chapter 2 that up to 70% of those in assisted living have some form of dementia or mental illness. So it is not unreasonable to say that many common emergencies in long-term care facilities are related to the fact that many residents have cognitive impairment so that those problems might be avoided by implementing specialized staff training to maximize the quality of care for residents with dementia. Anticipatory, preventive interventions are always preferable to emergency reactions and panicked responses.

Inadequate training is the single most significant factor resulting in poor or misguided care of the elderly, especially those with cognitive problems or dementia. Other than preventable behavior problems, what might be the ripple effect of the lack of caregivers' knowledge about aging and dementia? Staff (including management) will often presume that disruptive behaviors are inevitable in the progression of the disease. Such a presumption leads to the belief that there is little to do but to use tranquilizing medications to control the behavior. Frequently, the family is told that there are not enough staff caregivers to provide high levels of attention to residents and the families are then given the "option" of hiring privately paid caregivers to provide the extra help the resident needs. Of course, the unspoken message to family is that without either medication or private caregivers, the resident can no longer stay in the facility. Families who already feel overwhelmed and guilty about having to place their parent, spouse, or another relative with dementia in assisted living usually view the options as daunting and expensive. So they accept the status quo and hope for the best at the current facility, even though the care their loved one is receiving is of a considerably lesser quality than first promised.

Current Training Requirements

So what training are long-term care facilities required to provide their caregiver staff so they can anticipate problems and emergencies associated with dementia and intervene before they occur? You might think that state and/or federal regulations would put pressure on the long-term care industry to assure quality care. Think again!

The National Center for Assisted Living (NCAL) compiled information about regulations, including staff training, for assisted living facilities in all 50 states and the District of Columbia and reported that as of 2008, assisted living facilities in 12 states are not required to provide staff members who care for people with dementia with any specialized training over and above the general training expected of other employees in a long-term care or assisted living facility. [2] This means that in 12 states a caregiver without any extra training could be hired to work in a specialized unit for residents with dementia and behavior problems. In 18 states there is no specified training for non-specialty care assisted living staff regarding aging, dementia, behavior management, or mental illness. Yes, as shocking as it is, in these states direct-care staff are not required to have any training about the population they serve.

Even among states that currently have training requirements in place, the number of hours, type of training, training topics (curricula), and level of demonstrable knowledge vary widely. As an example of this variation in the training requirements across states, a person living in a long-term care or assisted living facility in Massachusetts will be cared for by a nursing aide who has had at least a 54-hour course of training, although Massachusetts only requires two hours of extra training to work in a dementia specialty care unit. The same resident living in a Delaware assisted living facility can be cared for by an aide who is not required to have any training at all. Delaware does not require training for staff in facilities that provide specialty care for those with dementia either. [2] So, in both states, the facilities meet the state requirements, but the training levels are certainly not comparable.

Furthermore, some states' regulations contain such vague statements as "trained to meet residents' needs," or "special training prior to resident contact," or "proper on-the-job training," which make it difficult to determine what training a caregiver has actually received. [2] These vaguely stated terms about training requirements invite a series of questions: What category of resident "need"? What kind of "special training"? What is considered "proper" on-the-job training?

Although some states specify the required content of training in assisted living, the topics may not include dementia or behavior management. For instance, New Mexico includes staff training topics such as fire safety, first aid, infection control, resident rights, and confidentiality of records. There are requirements to report abuse, neglect and exploitation, and to provide quality care "based on current resident needs." [2] While all of these are important general safety considerations,

New Mexico has no training specified for staff in dementia care units. Fire safety for residents with dementia would be very different from that required for cognitively intact elders, yet there is no recognition of this difference in the state-mandated training. Further, there is no indication that staff members are trained in the prevention of abuse and neglect of residents with dementia—again, a very different process than for cognitively intact elders. This is because persons with dementia often are not able to give coherent accounts of an event or even to report it.

Even in those states that outline mandatory requirements, regulations are sufficiently flexible that the type, quality, and to some extent, the amount of training offered can vary widely, depending on the priorities of the owners of a particular facility. Some owners are quite conscientious and might even offer additional training above that specified in the regulations, but others regard the requirements as mere check-off boxes to meet licensing requirements and do not devote sufficient time or energy to ensure that the training is meaningful.

If you are still unconvinced about the existence of a crisis in dementia care in assisted living, then consider the following facts. According to U.S. Department of Labor information [3]:

- A pet groomer usually has an apprenticeship of 6 to 10 weeks, meaning that the future groomer works with and is directly supervised by a licensed groomer before he or she can do the job alone. Fifty states have licensed grooming schools that provide training of 2 to 18 weeks' duration.

- A pest-control worker is usually required to have a high school diploma, and both federal and state laws require workers to be certified. In addition to general training in pesticide safety and use, state-required training usually involves 10 hours of classroom training and 60 hours of on-the-job training for each category of pest control work (e.g., rodents, fumigants, termites, turf). Even after training, workers must still be supervised until they have sufficient knowledge and experience to pass a certification test of knowledge and competency. Every 1 to 6 years, depending on the state, the worker must attend classes to become re-certified.

- A cosmetologist must have 9 to 24 months of training, and programs using an apprentice model can be 1 to 3 years in length.

That's right. The person who bathes and clips your dog, the person that sprays your home and even your lawn for bugs, and the person who styles your hair probably has considerably more training than the assisted living aide who provides care for your mother, your father, your aunt, your sister, or your friend in a dementia care unit. Indeed, considering that most training requirements for elder care are extremely meager, if you have read the information in Chapter 1 about brain function and behavior, you now know more than the majority of staff that take care of residents in dementia care facilities across the United States.

Continuing Education Requirements

Continuing education is a generally accepted way to keep up with new information and fine-tune one's job skills. However, according to the NCAL report, there are nine states that require no continuing education for caregivers in long-term care facilities. [2] Thirteen states require the administrators to have continuing education, and of those 13, only 7 states have any entity identified that would approve the education courses. In all, only 13 states have organizations empowered to approve the continuing education courses. In states that do have entities to approve continuing education, the approval is given by state licensing agencies rather than professional organizations. (Considering that most professional organizations for assisted living are actually trade organizations, even approval by such an oversight body might be prejudiced in favor of maximizing industry profits.) Otherwise, it is up to assisted living facilities to decide if their caregivers' training content is adequate. Among states with requirements for annual training in assisted living, the mandated number of training hours varies widely, from an unspecified number to more than 16. In many states, the required continuing education for caregiver staff who work in assisted living facilities is training "on dementia/cognitive impairment topics." A number of states require that the staff must have continuing education "specific to [the] population served" without any specification of the content of the curriculum or requirements for the different subgroups of the population. So there is no requirement stipulated for a higher level of training for caregivers in dementia units. Consider all this in an era when the incidence of dementia is exploding.

UNHEEDED CALL TO ACTION

Advocacy groups have called for a national long-term care standard, but their demands are vociferously opposed by the assisted living industry, which has strived to maintain the status quo even though the patchwork of state-by-state requirements is inadequate. What reasons would the long-term care industry have to maintain such a hodgepodge of regulations, while families remain in the dark about the skills of caregivers? Surely the industry leaders know that training in most of the business world is viewed as an investment in employees and is touted as a way to increase staff loyalty and assure clients' satisfaction. If the long-term care industry, assisted living in particular, is so dependent on maximizing their human resources, why does it see training as an "expense" rather than an investment? One clue comes from private conversations we have had with management who tell us that there is "no reason" to train such "low level" staff, because the turnover rate is so high. That is like saying there is no reason to educate children because a lot of them quit school before graduation.

Another reason for lack of training, we are told, is that the staff are not educated enough to understand something as complicated as the brain or behavior. If they are not educated enough to understand, then how can they be expected to care for our loved ones in the first place? And whose fault is it that they are not educated? In exploring the lack of appropriate training, we have become convinced that the assisted living industry views training as a cost while redecorating a facility, for example, is considered an investment. Training is such a low priority for some facilities that they refuse training even when it is offered to them at no cost! Of course, many such facilities truly believe and maintain that that they already provide training for their employees. However, as you now recognize, sometimes, the industry simply does not know how uneducated their employees really are about dementia. In addition, the very types of training offered currently in the industry do not address the real issues in dementia care, as you will see below.

Existing Training Models and Their Shortcomings

The long-term care training models that are most often used are as follows:

On-the-job training, whereby the new employees learn as they work, either by following a more experienced employee, or by informally asking questions of other caregivers with whom they come in contact. On-the-job training works well for teaching many skills. In dementia care, however, unless the more experienced "training" caregiver has a sufficiently developed level of knowledge and skill, a newcomer can be taught inappropriate interventions and ineffective skills through on-the-job training. The person passing on the knowledge must have sufficient expertise for the "on-the-job" training to be meaningful.

In-service training is offered during the workday; staff members are told to come to mandatory in-service training, which is usually on a payday. After the training session, the paychecks are handed out. Typically these sessions are very time-limited (45 minutes or so), which precludes going into much detail on complex topics such as dementia, behavior management, or psychiatric illnesses. All that staff members have to do is attend the session without necessarily being attentive, and given that (a) they have been coerced into coming in order to receive their paycheck, (b) they are often tired after a long shift, and (c) many have children and other pressing demands, who can blame them for not diving into the subject matter with gusto?

Ongoing training is a way of teaching the staff caregiver skills and imparting knowledge on a day-to-day basis as they work. This has some theoretical advantages, since the knowledge is likely to be directly applicable to the current work expected of the employee. However, in "ongoing training," the training staff have very little time to educate as they advise new employees about how to do tasks, because they also have to finish their own work. Most of us are familiar with this problem from our own experience. Haven't you said to yourself, "It's faster just to do it myself than to have to show someone else?" Well, this is precisely the shortcoming of ongoing training as a means of fulfilling training requirements. While it might have a place as part of a training curriculum, providing ongoing training is a very lengthy process, and information imparted on one occasion is less likely to be remembered and practiced on another occasion, later on, so it requires considerable educational skill in order to be effectively implemented.

Self-study training involves the use of workbooks, manuals, videos, and interactive computer programs to train employees. The idea is that caregivers' time is limited and not all caregivers can be scheduled at a certain time for a group training session. Therefore, it is much more convenient to provide a workbook or video that staff members can complete at their leisure. Most nurses and nurses' aides admit that this is the least effective training method of all. Directors of nursing have jokingly told us that they use training manuals as doorstops or paperweights. The trendy courses available online by computer offer some hope of better quality self-study, but currently are only minimally utilized due to perceived cost constraints. It will take a lot of convincing for assisted living facilities to spend money on training, when they continue to believe that dementia is adequately addressed with their present training.

Use of any of the common training models can save time, effort, and money and can provide the necessary hours of training required by the state and make the facility appear active in its effort to maintain a competent staff. In fact, there is nothing wrong with any of these models *per se*, but we are convinced that as they are currently utilized, they do not work well for adequately training caregivers in meeting the complex needs of residents with dementia. In dementia care, residents' behaviors change in response to medications, illnesses, the stage of disease and even the time of day, and so the skills of caregivers must be sufficiently sophisticated to allow them to respond adroitly to these challenges. The level of learning in many current models can be highly variable and inadequate, and thus the ability to apply the necessary skills to real-life caregiving situations is very limited.

We have decided, and others agree with us, that the assisted living facility staff and supervisors do not know what they do not know. They believe they have adequate training for the system in which they operate. Consequently if problems arise, they claim that it is the fault of the resident's dementia, not the lack of staff training. Problem behaviors are seen as a sign of the resident's dementia, not a sign of the result of staff ignorance. Take the following stories as examples of how lack of knowledge and training made things much worse than they had to be. As you read these, think about how you might have handled the situation, given that at this point you know more than most caregivers in long-term care.

Just Following Protocol: Negligence "by the Book" for Mrs. Addison

Mr. and Mrs. Addison moved into an assisted living facility when Mr. Addison, who had congestive heart failure, suffered a mild stroke. At home he had been having difficulty taking care of his wife, who had Alzheimer's disease. Subsequent to their move to the assisted living facility, Mr. Addison died and Mrs. Addison was alone without any assistance, so their son placed his mother in the facility's dementia care unit.

Over time, Mrs. Addison had more and more difficulty walking and keeping her balance. Because her disease prevented her from realizing, or understanding, that she had any problems, she would get up from her bed and try to go to the bathroom on her own. She fell on several occasions, and each time her son was called to drive her to the emergency room because she was on a blood thinner and her doctor wanted her to be thoroughly evaluated to rule out any problems. After Mrs. Addison's third fall, her son again found himself in the emergency room with his mother at almost the exact time as before and he began to wonder if there was more that the staff could do to prevent his mother's falls.

The staff at the dementia care unit tried to reassure him that they were monitoring his mother as best they could. They told him that they could not watch every resident 24 hours a day, and there was no way to prevent falls that occurred outside of their immediate supervision. They also said that his mother's daily routine was to nap after lunch and to be awakened by the staff before dinner. He was told that sometimes, though, his mother would get up from her nap and go into the bathroom on her own.

Putting the pieces together, Mrs. Addison's son realized that his mother's falls had occurred at the same time of day that the staff reported she sometimes got up on her own to go to the bathroom. However, when he mentioned to the staff that his mother had fallen at the same time of day on all three occasions, they did not seem to register this information as relevant to their caregiving. This disturbed Mrs. Addison's son, since even with the clear pattern to his mother's falls, the dementia care staff did not seem interested or inclined to work on a solution to the problem. He had expected that a dementia care unit would be attending to the behavior of the residents as a matter of routine. He was especially disturbed that when he brought problems to the staff, they seemed defensive and gave him the impression that they wanted him to lower his expectations for their care of his mother—almost as if repeated trips to the emergency room were no big deal. Mrs. Addison's son felt the staff's worst failing was that they had abandoned attempts to keep his mother as active as possible—a desire he had expressed from the beginning. In fact, his mother had usually been allowed to remain unattended in bed for most of the afternoon.

Of course, the thought of moving Mrs. Addison was almost more than her son could contemplate, so he finally offered a possible solution: Perhaps the staff could allow his mother to nap for an hour after lunch and then get her up to take her to the toilet. Fortunately, the staff at the facility was eager to make any changes that might help Mrs. Addison's quality of life, and so this reasonable solution was implemented—after which her afternoon falls ceased.

In this case, staff presumed that falls are part of Alzheimer's disease and cannot be controlled or monitored except with constant one-on-one supervision. It is true that as Alzheimer's disease progresses, physical ability decreases and the likelihood of falls increases. Chapter 1 explains how the brain controls our movements, balance, and how we see the world around us. As the disease progresses, so do the problems. Even so, there are often behavior patterns that go unrecognized unless someone takes the time to observe, review the facts, and deliberate. In the case of Mrs. Addison, a pattern that was obvious to her son was not even considered by the staff. If the staff had been trained to recognize and predict dementia-related behaviors rather than merely to follow protocols and rely on general knowledge, management of the environment and the risky situations could have been undertaken and the problem would have been solved.

Colonel Emerson: If You Yell, He'll Hear You

Mr. Emerson, an 85-year-old retired Air Force colonel, had lived in an assisted living community for about three years. Mr. Emerson had poor eyesight, which had been worsening significantly over the past few months. In addition, he was hard of hearing, but he did not like to wear his hearing aids because they picked up environmental noises that irritated him. Mr. Emerson also had cognitive problems and often forgot what he had been told by the staff.

Over time, the staff noticed that this previously pleasant gentleman was becoming paranoid, irritable, and very loud and agitated. Sometimes he would hit the staff when they tried to take care of him. The more they raised their voices to insist that he should be quiet, the angrier he became. Often, when the staff entered his room, he could not hear them when they mumbled that they were just checking on him, and when he would ask them what they were doing in his room, he could not hear the answer—he heard only a loud, unintelligible voice. This would make him angry because he thought the person was yelling at him. If he recognized the voice of a staff caregiver, he sometimes calmed down. However, if he could not recognize the caregiver, he would become even angrier. The staff dismissed a lot of his behavior as the "normal" worsening course of his dementia without considering how their own behavior affected his responses. They had been caring for and dealing with Mr. Emerson the same way for three years and had not considered that his decline called for a new way of interacting with him.

By now, you will recognize that adequate training about aging could have helped the situation with Colonel Emerson. Sensory losses, especially hearing and vision, are particularly difficult burdens for an individual whose brain cannot process information. In addition, sensory losses can contribute to depression, which may be exhibited as irritability and social isolation.

Remember that the brain affects how we express our feelings, and the brain of a person with cognitive impairment does not appropriately respond in emotional situations. Sometimes, behavioral changes are the earliest signs of physical problems such as visual or hearing loss. In these cases, the environment and staff behaviors can be modified to make a resident's life more fulfilling and dignified. This example also points out the importance of regular re-evaluation of residents by a multidisciplinary team that is knowledgeable about brain function.

Mr. Alvin: His "Cup Runneth Over"

Mr. Alvin had dementia, and he was often very confused and tearful. When he was transferred to the dementia care unit of the long-term care facility where he lived, he could not understand why he had to live "at this place" or eat with all "those old people." Because Mr. Alvin had fallen so many times when he got up out of bed to use the toilet at night, and because he tended to become disoriented during the night and urinate in the corner of the room, a urinal was placed on his nightstand for him to use. Although he did use the urinal, he would then promptly pour it out next to the bed.

The staff repeatedly reprimanded him when, each morning, they found he had dumped the contents of his urinal, and they had had long discussions with him about the need to be clean and obedient. Each time, Mr. Alvin, having completely forgotten what he had done the night before, would become angry and accuse the staff of making up stories about him. His behavior escalated to the point that he constantly complained about the way his room smelled, the bad food, the rude staff, and that there was nothing interesting to do. The staff liked him less and less and began and began to complain to each other about his behavior. Most of the aides believed that Mr. Alvin was trying to make them look bad and irritate them for fun. If his call light came on, a sigh or slight moan would go up from the aides, some of whom would look around for someone else to go to his room.

After several months, the director of the facility called Mr. Alvin's psychiatrist and told her that Mr. Alvin was a very difficult resident despite the staff's having tried "everything" to control his behavior. The director asked the psychiatrist whether she could put him on a medicine that would make him obey them. As it turned out, there was a medication that helped Mr. Alvin "behave," but in addition, the psychiatrist educated the staff about the fact that Mr. Alvin was not intentionally trying to anger them. She recommended that the staff look for positive ways to interact with Mr. Alvin outside traditional care activities. After that, he stopped dumping his urinal, and he sometimes even called for help when he needed to go to the bathroom.

A month went by, and the same psychiatrist was called about a problem with another resident. When she arrived at the facility, an aide was talking to Mr. Alvin in the hallway, and they were laughing. The psychiatrist heard a new staff member say, "He's such a nice man."

What happened in this case was that Mr. Alvin's dementia interfered with (1) his ability to remember what happened the night before and (2) his ability to comprehend the consequences of his actions. Because the staff reprimanded him about things he did not remember, he became suspicious and cross. The staff, who mistakenly believed his behavior was intentional, in turn became irritated with him much of the time, and that attitude further exacerbated Mr. Alvin's unhappiness. Once he stopped dumping his urinal, the staff began to relax and did not dread spending time with him. They stopped reprimanding Mr. Alvin and began to have more positive interactions with him. In turn, there were fewer complaints from him, so staff members were more likely to have conversations with him.

In this situation, the combination of a judicious use of medication and changes in staff behaviors were successful in leading to a positive solution. This is an important point, because many people mistakenly believe that, since dementia is a disease that progresses, medications are the only means to control behavior problems. This lack of awareness and understanding is the reason why direct care workers do not receive the training they need. Conversely, some people believe that any medication intervention for behavior disturbances is irresponsible.

Had this staff known about dementia and the way

that dysfunction of the frontal lobes affects behavior, they could have focused specifically on Mr. Alvin's urinal-dumping behavior problem rather than interpreting all of his behavior as a personal attack. They also could have called the psychiatrist much earlier, before things got so difficult. In the meantime, they could have been interacting with Mr. Alvin in a more pleasant, dignified way, resulting in more positive behaviors from him.

THE CRYING NEED FOR EFFECTIVE TRAINING STRATEGIES

Too often, training is a "rubber stamp" process in order to meet guidelines and regulations. In our professional roles working with people with dementia, it has become clear to us that most assisted living facilities consider training of caretaker staff a problem or an obstacle because the facility has to juggle resident care with the number of staff employed, the number on duty at any one shift, and budgetary constraints. This perspective can lead to benign—sometimes egregious—neglect of proper training of employees in caregiver jobs. This is not to say that there are not very gifted caregivers in assisted living, as well as extremely well-run facilities, but based on our experience, these gifted caregivers are often unable to explain why they are successful with patients and residents. Much of the time they believe their success stems from their likability or personality. In essence, this speaks to their lack of knowledge, understanding, and training in effective care strategies.

The type of training that appears to be the most effective is that which includes interactive (with role-play) presentation of actual or representative care situations, active problem solving in small groups, and detailed discussions. There are a number of models of adult learning available for learners of all educational backgrounds, so that the level of education of a caregiver should not be an obstacle to teaching important principles and skills. This approach to education takes time—more time than a one-hour lecture or a quick review of basic skills—but obviously, it is also a better investment.

Efforts have been made to address the problems in training; some have been more successful than others. Such efforts (primarily nursing homes and adult day care) include the Wellspring model in nursing home care [4], Resident-Assisted Montessori Programming (RAMP) [5], and the Center for Nursing and Rehabilitation Peer Mentoring program. [6] One factor in these models that appears to be important in the transfer of knowledge from training to job performance is instructor assistance on-site at the facility on a regular basis, so education can occur as soon as behavior management problems arise. In this model, staff members have access to an expert who can guide them to change their approaches to residents, change the environment, or work with management on policies. Regrettably, it is rare that facilities have the benefit of such individuals in their midst.

The Alzheimer's Association offers a choice of classroom or online training in six areas to direct care workers and other facility staff who are involved in care. [7] The training guidelines are based, according to the Association, on a review of research regarding successful management strategies for pain management, food and fluid consumption, social engagement, wandering, falls, and restraint-free care. [8, 9] However, reviewers were clear that behavior management strategies need to be tailored to the individual's needs and abilities. Whether the Alzheimer's training programs are effective remains to be seen since the training may be provided by Association staffers who have not worked with individuals with dementia, have not provided services in long-term care settings, or are unaware of staffing issues in assisted living. It seems to us that training in how to determine the needs of the individual, understand how dementia affects those needs, and analyze patterns of behavior in the individual would be more effective than simple guidelines for management of the six behavioral areas. A great deal of time, effort, and money has gone into the careful development of this program, so we expect that ongoing surveys of the effectiveness of the Alzheimer's Association training will be forthcoming and will provide more information upon which to build additional effective and efficient training programs.

Another tactic used to maximize training is to provide that training as part of a research program. Researchers in academic settings can obtain grant funding for studies on the effectiveness of a training paradigm or a new approach to teaching a concept, and then offer the services at long-term care facilities at no direct cost to the facility. The facility receives free training services and also gets recognition, which improves marketing. While this may seem at first glance to be a win-win situation, the issue is that research processes are very different from day-to-day operations. In addition, with the research directors heavily involved in the day-to-day functioning of the caregivers, there is an automatic improvement in caregiver performance, but after the research project is over, what process is in place to maintain these benefits?

Here are our questions:

1. If there are existing programs that have already stood the test of time and shown increases in quality care, reductions in staff turnover, and increases in overall

satisfaction for both staff and residents, then why are they not widely used?

2. Why has there not been an immediate adoption of the processes of these programs in nursing homes and assisted living facilities?

Consider this: Assisted living is a competitive business in which each company must be unique and also demonstrate its comparative excellence. Each facility in each town has to discern the factors potential residents consider when choosing a residence: Are they staff training, furnishings, room size, cost, location, or a combination of these? Then they must strive to be the absolute best. Consumers must make it clear to the long-term care industry that emphasis on training—and, therefore, the quality of care—are the prime factors in they consider when weighing their options. Training and quality of care must supersede considerations such as how nice a residence looks, or even its location. Until families and residents demand a certain level of training from all of assisted living, there will continue to be a focus on physical amenities and prices rather than true quality care.

References

1. King, Marsha. Providers fighting assisted-living rules that would raise standards. *Seattle Times* September 8, 2003.

2. The National Center for Assisted Living. Assisted living state regulatory review (March 2008). Available at: www. ncal.org/about/state_review.cfm; accessed March 15, 2009.

3. U.S. Department of Labor. Occupational Outlook Handbook, 2008-2009 Ed. Available at: www.bls.gov/oco/ocos254.htm; accessed August 2008.

4. Stone, Robyn I, Reinhard, Susan C, Bowers, B, et al. Re-evaluation of the Wellspring model for improving nursing home quality (for the Commonwealth Fund, August 2002). Available at: www.wellspringis.org/index.html; accessed August 2008.

5. Camp, CJ, and Skrajner, MJ. Resident-Assisted Montessori Programming (RAMP): Training persons with dementia to serve as group activity leaders. *The Gerontologist* 2004;44(3):426-431.

6. National Clearinghouse on the Direct Care Workforce. Available at: www.directcareclearinghouse.org/practices; accessed August 2008.

7. Alzheimer's Association. Available at: www.alz.org/professionals_and_researchers_11176.asp; accessed July 17, 2008.

8. Tilly, J, and Reed, P. Evidence on Interventions to Improve Quality of Care for Residents with Dementia in Assisted Living and Nursing Homes. Chicago, IL: Alzheimer's Association, 2004.

9. Tilly, J, and Reed, P. Falls, Wandering and Physical Restraints: Interventions for Residents with Dementia in Assisted Living and Nursing Homes. Chicago, IL: Alzheimer's Association, 2006. Available at www.alz.org

CHAPTER FOUR
THE "CULTURE CHANGE" MOVEMENT

Mrs. Addison: Bah Humbug

Christmas was in five days, and Mrs. Addison's son went to visit her in the dementia care facility. The environment was very homey, with an open floor plan. The door to each resident's room opened out to a spacious living and dining area, where staff could easily keep track of the whereabouts and activities of all the residents. Because Mrs. Addison had a tendency to attempt getting up out of bed on her own, her bed was moved closer to the door, so the nursing staff could easily keep watch on her while she rested or reach her quickly if the bed alarm indicated she was trying to get out of bed.

When he approached her room, Mrs. Addison's son was immediately met with green and silver tinsel garland draping her door frame, along with small shiny ornaments hanging from it. Upon entering the room, he found the same garland wrapped around every picture frame (again with small shiny ornaments) and inventively paired with small colored lights along the bottom of the window frame near his mother's bed.

The furniture had been rearranged, so his mother's bed was against the back wall away from the door. On the small table at the end of her bed, instead of the family photographs she was used to, there was a lighted, decorated artificial Christmas tree. Under it was draped a tree skirt, and on top of the skirt stood a large stuffed dog and a doll dressed as an angel. The aide on duty excitedly pointed out the decorations and gifts left by another aide.

The longer her son visited, the more apparent if became that Mrs. Addison believed the new things in her room did not belong to her. Furthermore, she no longer recognized her own furniture. She even rejected the gift of Christmas candy sent by a dear relative, because she did not believe it was hers. No amount of persuasive effort was successful in convincing her otherwise.

Over the next two days, Mrs. Addison became increasingly irritated and anxious, and when her son mentioned the tree and the lights, she would say, "When are they coming to get these? Where is that dog going to stay? Who's going to take care of the dog?" When an aide came in and cheerfully said, "Are you ready for Christmas?" Mrs. Addison looked shocked. Then, with a worried countenance, she said, "What? I have to get things done!" Turning to her son, she said, "Did you know about this?"

Her son decided to remove the decorations and the toy dog. He instructed the staff to keep the tree lights off. At this point the staff began to apologize when they saw him, emphasizing that the aide should have gotten the family's permission to redecorate the room. Of course, he knew the aide's heart had been in the right place and that she had just wanted her favorite resident to have a happy holiday. Unfortunately, the aide's lack of knowledge about his mother's attitude toward holidays, and her need for familiar surroundings, had resulted in distress rather than joy. What happened?

A major part of dementia care is knowledge about the person–the past experiences, the personality quirks, the things that are considered a responsibility rather than a joy. Had the staff asked the family (and even Mrs. Addison) how she had experienced Christmas in the past, they would have realized that for Mrs. Addison, Christmas represented a time of pressure and stress instead of a joyful time to be shared. All her adult life, Mrs. Addison had struggled throughout the Christmas season to entertain and accomplish the myriad tasks necessary to make others happy. In fact, recognizing this, in the past few years, Mrs. Addison had stopped decorating because with her advancing age, decorations were not considered a necessity, but were viewed as frivolous objects that heralded chaotic gatherings and guilt about not being able to take charge of dinners and gifts as she had in the past. She preferred not to be reminded.

In addition to ignoring Mrs. Addison's personal history, the staff did not consider that dementia makes it difficult for anyone to adapt to new surroundings, new people, or new objects, even if the new objects are in one's own room. Although natural, it was erroneous for the staff to consider their own experiences to be universal and presume that all residents need decorations and reminders of the upcoming holidays. Yes, it was generous and caring that Mrs. Addison was treated as a person and not a disease by the aide who had lovingly decorated the room. However, in this case, neither the person nor the disease was considered in her treatment. Of course, the ignorance was not the fault of the aide, but the fault of the training system in the assisted living facility.

In this chapter you will learn about the terms Culture Change and Person-Centered Care that have woven their way into the language of long-term care, especially assisted living. As you learn more about these concepts, think about Mrs. Addison and how true Person-Centered Care would have prevented her bad Christmas experience.

DE-INSTITUTIONALIZATION OF LONG-TERM CARE

No one relishes the idea of living in a nursing home. It is generally accepted that most people, if given the choice, would rather stay in their own homes rather than go to a nursing home. When most people think of nursing homes, they envision an emotionally cold warehouse with old people sitting in wheelchairs lined up against the wall for hours at a time, bathed and fed against their will. Nursing homes were based on a disease care model (like a hospital—forever): If one needed help, one pushed a call button and a nurse would come. People were "treated" with medications and bed rest. Such an environment is not appealing to residents, families, or caregivers.

Since the 1970's, there has been an attempt to de-institutionalize long-term care. This approach was referred to as humanistic [1], in which the focus of care is the humanity of the residents rather than task-oriented institutional regimentation. Culture Change was born from the notion that regardless of a person's condition, his or her dignity should be maintained, the surroundings in which he or she lived should be comforting rather than distressing, and caregivers should be viewed as trusted allies rather than automatons focused on a task. The aim was that elders, rather than being warehoused in an institution, would be cared for in a home-like environment. Like living at "home," the resident would have a voice in the process of his or her own care. The ability to make choices about food, bath times, bedtimes, and even where to sit in the dining room would help to maintain the person's dignity and sense of humanity.

Besides being intuitively obvious, scientific studies have shown that care is improved when the resident is allowed to have more control. [2]

Although the idea has been around since the 1970's, Culture Change is now considered a revolution in long-term care. With the revolution, there have been significant changes in the way care is provided in nursing homes, resulting in residents feeling less helpless and less bored. [3] Changing the nursing home environment makes sense, of course. To de-institutionalize such a setting seems obvious. Essentially, the culture of the nursing home would change to be more humanistic and more home-like. Assisted living hasn't been left out of the revolution: In the new "Culture Change" enthusiasm, even the term assisted living facility (ALF) has come under fire for sounding too institutional. Several less offensive options have been tried, such as assisted living residence (ALR) or assisted living community (ALC). With Culture Change, the term unit (where a number of residents live on a common hallway) has become the "neighborhood."

But wait—wasn't assisted living itself supposed to change the way assistance and care is provided to elders? Well, remember that despite the original intent of assisted living—that is, aging in place (see Chapter 2)—the assisted living facility now looks similar to a nursing home. What began as a place for ambulatory, active seniors who often could still drive but needed a little help (like the ones in the ads), assisted living facilities have turned into a place where wheelchairs, walkers, medication carts, and private nurses abound. Rather quickly, the assisted living model has become the "Mini-Me" of nursing homes, with 50% to 70% of the residents having some form of dementia.

Person-Centered Care: The Next Hot Thing

Other terms, such as resident-centered or person-centered, have woven their way into the language of long-term care, especially assisted living, and have been used to convey the same concept as Culture Change. It has been difficult at times to differentiate the term Culture Change from Person-Centered care; indeed, industry experts often use the terms interchangeably. It seems that Culture Change connotes the appearance of a facility (home-like), the way the staff interact with the residents (with dignity), and some policies and procedures (broader mealtime schedules).

What is really meant by the concept of Person-Centered approach? In our online article [4], we try to explain:

> Perhaps the best way to view Person-Centered Care is to imagine how you would expect care of an elderly resident to look if that resident were your own family member. You would take into account personality factors, personal history, and knowledge of likes and dislikes. This information would be based on your longstanding relationship with the person and your knowledge of their idiosyncratic patterns of behavior. So, of course, you would use that knowledge when you approached the person, when you spoke to them, when you touched them, when you engaged in activities with them, and when you talked about them with others.

The presumption that a caregiver would be more understanding and empathic if he or she was aware of the resident's past experiences has been borne out in research. [5] But does Culture Change equal Person-Centered care? Perhaps the next story will help illustrate:

Mrs. Smith: Under Attack

Mrs. Smith, a generally kind 80-year-old lady, had lived in a dementia care community for only a short time. In conformance to the new "Culture Change" philosophy of the community, her biography was placed in a wall-mounted "memory box" next to her room so that others could know her background and her interests. Very soon after she moved into the facility, the formerly good-natured lady began to display combativeness and agitation. Not all of the aides had observed this behavior, but after word spread among them, they realized that the Filipino aide and the Korean nurse were the main targets of Mrs. Smith's ire. She would accuse them of being spies and traitors and refuse to let them take care of her. Often she would yell at them to leave her room and leave her alone.

Because of the facility's general policy of dealing directly and swiftly with any hint of "racism" or racist acts, and because the Korean nurse and Filipino aide felt insulted, the nursing director had many long talks with Mrs. Smith during which she explained in great detail that Mrs. Smith needed to be more tolerant of other people and that racism was a zero tolerance issue in the community. During these sessions, Mrs. Smith acted embarrassed and expressed complete agreement with the director of nursing. She would say she was sorry that she had hurt anyone's feelings, and of course she wasn't racist. However, even immediately after one of these talks, if the Filipino aide entered her room, Mrs.

Smith would begin to yell for help and tell her to get out. After these episodes, it was difficult to calm Mrs. Smith, and she would make comments about the "danger" that was "everywhere."

A psychiatric evaluation of Mrs. Smith was obtained. In his evaluation, the psychiatrist found some interesting information that had not been conveyed to him in the initial consultation request. The staff at the dementia care facility called Mrs. Smith "Colonel" because she had been a career U.S. Army nurse. During World War II she had seen many combat situations during her assignment in the Pacific theater and had been briefly held as a prisoner by the Japanese just prior to the end of the war. When the doctor talked to her about her experiences, Mrs. Smith became tearful and discussed how afraid she had been for her life, especially when she was imprisoned. Evidently, she had been able to suppress the combat memories for many years. She stated that "now the Japanese were back" and claimed they were again holding her prisoner. Her comments to the psychiatrist revealed that she interpreted the secured facility as a prison, viewed the Filipino aide and the Korean nurse as her captors, and thought the other staff and the residents were prisoners like herself.

The facility administration's solution was to transfer the Filipino aide and the Korean nurse out of the unit to another part of the facility. The two had been very effective and knowledgeable staff members, but they were nevertheless transferred without any attempt to solve the real problem because of the staff's lack of understanding about how dementia affects the brain and how to use Culture Change to provide Person-Centered care.

In addition to memory boxes, a new culture-change trend in caring for the elderly is to place resident biographies at the entrance of his or her room, especially in a dementia care community. This is done to provide others with a personal profile of the resident so that others can appreciate the full lives the resident led prior to the onset of the dementia, rather than defining the residents in terms of their disease. The posting of theses personal profiles facilitates the staff's understanding the roots of the resident's behavior. For instance, if a resident had been the CEO of a major corporation, the staff's approach to that person might be different than their approach to someone whose career provided less authority over others.

Such biographical information is a great idea. However, staff may not take time to read the biographies, and sometimes, staff's reading abilities are so low that such biographical information is too difficult for them. We have had the experience of staff's asking us to put biographies on video so that they could participate since they were unable to read the biographies provided. Frequently, even if they do read the biographical information, poorly trained staff members do not place a resident's behavior in the context of those biographies. The case of Mrs. Smith is a good example of staff's lack of association between past experiences and current behavior in people with dementia. War experiences, because they are so traumatic, can lead to bad memories even in older individuals without dementia. Because dementia affects one's information-processing abilities and memory, the individual can feel as if he or she is living in the past. In the case of Mrs. Smith, all the staff knew was that she had been an Army nurse, even though her full biography was there for all to read. No one connected the facts about Mrs. Smith's wartime experiences in the Pacific with the possibility that an Asian face might, for her, be a strong negative stimulus, bringing back some horrible memories.

How else could the staff have been more effective? Individuals with dementia are often unable to understand the situation in which they currently find themselves— that is, living in assisted living facilities—because they are not aware that they have any problems. They may admit to some memory failings, but they believe that they can still live independently. This is because a part of the brain called the frontal lobes is affected by the disease. The frontal lobes of a person with dementia do not work very well in real-life situations, in which processing must take place very quickly. This is why reasoning with a person with dementia does not result in behavior change. Their behavior is not based on a thoughtful plan or logical evaluation of facts or situations; rather, it is based on reactions to the world as they see it at that moment. Thus, when the problem was described to her, Mrs. Smith understood that yelling at someone was not appropriate. However, in the real situation, her frontal lobes did not function properly to prevent her inappropriate behavior. Because the frontal lobe dysfunction caused by dementia results in a person's being less able to prevent unwanted behavior (referred to as *disinhibition*), a person with dementia may make comments that seem racist or biased, even though such behavior is totally uncharacteristic for the individual.

To solve this problem, techniques could have been used to reduce the "meaning" or "identity" (spies and captors) that Mrs. Smith associated with the Asian staff. For example, in order to neutralize the situation, all the staff could have been asked to wear American flag pins, or the Filipino aide and her Korean colleague could have worn a badge that said "Proud to be an American." They could have been asked to interact with Mrs. Smith at times that did not require any care, such as in a fun activity or at mealtime, thus building more rapport. The staff could sing patriotic songs during group activities, with the Filipino aide helping to lead the singing. Over time, Mrs. Smith might be more accepting of the aide and the nurse. Remember that the purpose of Culture Change and Person-Centered care is to form a trusting, calming relationship between caregiver and resident. Clearly, this was not attempted in Mrs. Smith's case.

The following is another example of Person-Centered care without the proper understanding of how the disease affects behavior. Indeed, many agree that one of the crucial aspects of implementing Person-Centered care in a specialty dementia care facility is training staff about dementia. [6]

Mrs. Hawkins: "Anorexia"

Poor Mrs. Hawkins had not been eating. She would go to the dining room, a spacious room with elegantly set tables, but would come to a complete stop at the dining room threshold. The staff would have to take her by the arm, lead her to her table, and convince her to sit down. Sometimes they would be in a hurry, so they would take her by the shoulders and try to place her in the chair. She would not speak and would look fearful, then would bolt from the dining room, mumbling and covering her ears. The staff could not convince Mrs. Hawkins to eat the food, and she could say only, "I must not be hungry."

The director of the facility reported to Mrs. Hawkins'

grandson that she was not eating. Thinking she might not like the food, her grandson began to bring her food from restaurants in order to get her to eat and he began sitting with her in the dining room at mealtimes. Even he had difficulty keeping her at the table. Soon, Mrs. Hawkins became extremely anxious all the time and was referred to a psychologist for "counseling" about her anxiety and to find out why she would not eat. The staff was perplexed, and no one could give much information except to say, "She's been that way for a long time."

Because Mrs. Hawkins could not report her feelings very well to the psychologist, he decided to observe her at mealtime to find out what was going on. He noticed that the dining room staff was jovial but did not engage the residents in much conversation. They would hurry from kitchen to table, often calling loudly to each other to ask about the availability of a certain dish or for help busing the tables. When Mrs. Hawkins appeared at the dining room threshold and came to a stop, she seemed afraid. Her eyes got big and her mouth opened wide. A couple of times she glanced furtively from side to side, but mostly she looked down. Any noise seemed to startle her, and the joviality of the servers seemed to annoy her and make her anxious. When at her table, she kept her head down. One of her tablemates apparently could not hear well, and she would yell out whatever she needed, like, "Where's salt?" or "What's this stuff here?" Mrs. Hawkins then would startle and look fearfully at the woman. The psychologist quickly discerned that the underlying cause of Mrs. Hawkins' anxiety was the fact that because of her brain dysfunction, she was unable to interpret the noises around her as friendly, animated conversation or loud *questions, and she had difficulty understanding what others were saying, especially with the background noise in the dining room.*

The psychologist asked the director of the facility if Mrs. Hawkins could be allowed to eat in her room. He was told that the policies of the facility would not allow this because she might choke or hurt herself with utensils and the staff had to be able to see everyone eating. What about eating in a quieter area, perhaps with an aide that could eat at the same time with Mrs. Hawkins? The facility director said that was impossible, because they needed all the aides to be in the dining room, and aides were not allowed to eat while the residents ate. The director took it upon herself to eat with Mrs. Hawkins in the main office. However, because of the administrator's open door policy and need for confidentiality with families, this became unsatisfactory. Besides, Mrs. Hawkins would become disturbed and distracted by people coming and going, asking questions, or laughing at things she did not understand.

Rules and regulations do not take into account the need for flexibility with residents with dementia. Noise, loud talking, and large areas can confuse a person with dementia, resulting in lack of appetite, sleep disturbance, refusing help, or self-isolation. A dining room that a person with normal brain function would perceive as pleasantly spacious may be perceived as threatening by a person with dementia. How much simpler for Mrs. Hawkins, the staff, and Mrs. Hawkins's family if the dementia unit staff had only understood how a dysfunctional brain processes noises and language. They would have known they needed to reduce the noise in her surroundings and would have been aware that loud talking upset her.

One simple culture-change solution would have been to have Mrs. Hawkins eat at a different time, when there would be fewer people in the dining room. Another option would have been to tailor the facility's policies to such situations, so that Mrs. Hawkins could eat in a smaller, quieter area while an aide ate a meal as well. The goal is for mealtime to become a calmer experience, leading to less anxious, less agitated, better nourished residents. In a pleasant, calm and interactive environment, the staff is likely to be more aware of changes in appetite or behavior that might signal other important problems for the residents.

MISAPPLICATION OF "PERSON-CENTERED" TO DEMENTIA CARE

Recognizing such situations and modifying the environment to accommodate residents with dementia should be the true goal of Culture Change. Consider why persons with dementia are placed in a facility. They are unable to care for themselves, and their behavior may be such that they refuse care because they are unaware that they have problems that need care in the first place. Additionally, judgment is impaired in people with dementia, and behavior problems may interfere with personal relationships. If the person with dementia were able to plan his or her own schedule, actively participate in care, and maintain as much independence as possible, why would he or she require placement in a dementia care facility? The appropriate provision of dementia care, we argue, is defined by knowing the patient's patterns of behavior, understanding how the brain disease affect those patterns, and focusing on the

81

immediate needs of the resident rather than the facility schedules. It is redundant to use the terms Person-Centered care and dementia care together. If facility staff are professing that they are changing their approach to Person-Centered dementia care, then what kind of care were they providing before?

DOES PERSON-CENTERED CARE EQUAL KNOWLEDGE?

Some have said that the person should be treated, not the disease. [7] Laudable as this sounds, this is not completely true for dementia care, because the disease affects the person. Knowledge about aging, especially dementia, is necessary when one provides services to elders. Some have said that the person should be treated, not the disease. [7] Laudable as this sounds, it is not completely true for dementia care, because the disease affects the person. It is not enough to have compassion and sympathy. Remember Mrs. Addison's situation? As the stories in this chapter illustrate, a caregiver must be able to synthesize the personal information about the resident with knowledge about the disease. The caregiver must know someone's personal history, understand how dementia affects the brain and how the diseased brain can change behavior, and then use that knowledge to provide care that meets the needs of the resident in a compassionate and dignified way.

Caring without knowledge can be as harmful as knowledge without caring. What is lacking from the Culture Change movement is the increase in knowledge about the brain of the person one is caring for. It is not enough for a caregiver in an assisted living or other long-term care facility to stop using words like "the Alzheimer's patient in room 102B" and start referring to the person by name. Can you not include the disease in your knowledge of the resident? The disease changes the person's behavior, and, in turn, changes the needs and desires. The person's history is an important aspect of care, whether or not the person can accurately recall it, or even in the case that they are overly focused on it. However, understanding the person's history should be integrated with an understanding of how that person is affected by dementia.

DOES PERSON-CENTERED CARE EQUAL QUALITY CARE?

Quality care is a concept that is frequently brought up but not easily defined. If quality care in general is difficult to define and to quantify, then quality dementia care is even more problematic. For instance, quality care to increase one's sense of autonomy in assisted living would mean allowing any resident to leave the facility at will. However, such freedom would not constitute quality care for a resident with dementia. Indeed, the ability of a person with Alzheimer's or another form of dementia to leave the facility at will could be considered negligence on the part of the facility in certain circumstances.

WHAT YOU CAN DO TO HELP ENSURE TRUE PERSON-CENTERED CARE

In assisted living, one could argue that Person-Centered care and Culture Change are just different terms for customer service. An Internet search for the definition of customer service results in common threads. In essence, customer service means that a business provides a service or a product based on the customer's needs or desires and implies that the business does not make promises it cannot keep. Sound familiar? The reader might be interested to know that the term Culture Change is being used in businesses other than long-term care. Indeed, it has probably been in use longer than in these other industries.

So what is a consumer to do? Don't become enchanted by the marketing ploy of the buzzword Person-Centered care. If it does not equal more knowledge or true quality care, then it is simply a rephrasing of customer service. If consumers enter a facility that proudly states in its literature, "We provide Person-Centered care," and this is echoed by the facility's marketing staff and administration, ask when, where, and how. The answers may be surprising.

Besides, the term Person-Centered care really begs important questions: Why must the staff be trained to be friendly with residents, when the main mission of the facility is to provide service and care? What have residents and families been paying for, if not service, a home-like setting, and the ability to maintain as much independence as possible?

What if Culture Change and Person-Centered care were combined with increased knowledge about how the brain works, how dementia affects brain function, and how behaviors are changed when such a disease is now part of the person? Increased knowledge of brain-behavior relationships does not mean that one has to abandon a Person-Centered approach. We would argue that it enhances one's ability to understand the person and ultimately leads to the best quality of care that can be provided. Until families and residents ask questions and expect to be active participants in care of their loved one, the system will be the same regardless of the culture of the assisted living or other long-term care facility—neither the person nor dementia as a disease will be the focus of care.

REFERENCES

1. Tobin, Sheldon S. "The Historical Context of 'Humanistic' Culture Change in Long-Term Care." in *Culture Change in Long-Term Care.* eds. Audrey S. Weiner and Judah L. Ronch (Philadelphia: Haworth Press, 2003), pp. 53-64.

2. Werezak, Leona J, and Morgan, Debra G. Creating a therapeutic psychosocial environment in dementia care: a preliminary framework. *Journal of Gerontological Nursing* 2003;29(12):18-25.

3. Bergman-Evans, Brenda. Beyond the basics: effects of the Eden alternative model on quality of life issues. *Journal of Gerontological Nursing* 2004;30(6):7-34.

4. Goethe, KE, and Leatherman, ME. Can person-centered care be saved? *Long-Term Living Magazine.* Posted online May 1, 2009: http://tinyurl.com/dyf5xd or www.ltlmagazine.com

5. Rasin, Joyce, and Kautz, Donald D. Knowing the resident with dementia: perspectives of assisted living facility caregivers. *Journal of Gerontological Nursing* 2007;33(69):30-36.

6. Gnaedinger, Nancy. "Changes in Long-Term Care for Elderly People with Dementia: A Report from the Front Lines in British Columbia, Canada." in *Culture Change in Long-Term Care.* eds. Audrey S. Weiner and Judah L. Ronch (Philadelphia: Haworth Press, 2003), pp. 355-371

7. Kitwood, Tom. *Dementia Reconsidered: The Person Comes First.* Maidenhead, Berkshire, UK: Open University Press, 1997.

CHAPTER FIVE
THE HOSPICE "SOLUTION"

There has been a recent surge of effort to educate the public and healthcare providers about end-of-life care. This effort has been very successful and has helped thousands of terminally ill people and their families. Comfort that had been neglected as medicine became more technologically advanced has re-emerged as the focus of caring for those with incurable illness. However, as you will see in this chapter, one problem is that hospice often becomes *de facto* end-of-life care for Alzheimer's disease when other interventions might be more appropriate.

HOSPICE VERSUS END-OF-LIFE CARE

Early on, hospice was a way to help the dying in a way that assured comfort and dignity. Later, people started using terms like "palliative care" and "end-of-life care," and over time, these terms became interchangeable, even in guidelines promulgated by national agencies. However, hospice care and palliative care can actually be different care models. Palliative care is designed to provide wide-ranging physical, emotional, and spiritual care for patients at any time during a life-threatening illness.

According to the World Health Organization, among other things, palliative care "is applicable early in the course of illness, in conjunction with other therapies that are intended to prolong life, such as chemotherapy or radiation therapy . . .." [1] This means that palliative care is not incompatible with treatment of the primary and terminal condition, although most commonly, a person being given palliative care does not have the primary terminal condition treated. So, for example, a patient with severe emphysema that was expected to lead to death could receive palliative care which could include treatment designed to treat the emphysema (primary or terminal condition), even though it was not expected to "cure" the disease. Most often such a patient receiving palliative care would receive no treatment for the primary disease, but would receive treatment for other conditions. So, for example, he would not necessarily go to the hospital every time he became short of breath. Instead, comfort measures such as narcotics might be given, although if he developed a complication of his emphysema such as pneumonia, he might be treated with antibiotics although the antibiotic treatment would not be expected to affect his underlying, primary condition which is emphysema. In that sense, palliative care is a broader term than hospice care, but the two terms are often confused. When considering palliative care, it is important to remember that elders with chronic debilitating illnesses can receive appropriate and compassionate end-of-life care without the intervention of hospice—after all, people have been caring for loved ones at the end of life without a formal "hospice" model for centuries, and physicians were caring for dying housebound patients long before anyone thought to give such care a special name. During the 20th Century, health care advanced in industrialized countries in such a way that the process of dying became more detached from the family. The palliative care movement appropriately re-focused attention on providing humane comfort care for those with chronic incurable illness. The focus of care moved from comforting the dying to heroic interventions in order to prolong lives. However, that does not mean that the art of caring for terminal patients was universally lost to caregivers—either professional or lay.

In contrast to palliative care, hospice care is a formalized model that does not attempt to reverse, improve, or impact the terminal condition based on the expectation that the patient will die within six months. While it incorporates components of palliative care (e.g. comfort measures, spiritual and emotional support) the care is specifically given at the end of life. So, while there is overlap, and although the field is evolving, palliative care and hospice care are not always synonymous.

When we think of hospice, most of us have in mind a small group of volunteers who freely give of their time and resources to help the dying. That was true about 30 years ago, but hospice has increasingly become very big business because hospice care has linked into the health care entitlement system so that Medicare and Medicaid now pay for end-of-life care in a structured and formalized way when it is provided through hospice, rather than paying for individual services provided piecemeal to dying patients outside a hospice "package." According to a RAND study from 2004, the use of hospice services has changed dramatically since Medicare first began paying for hospice benefits in the late 1980's. Since that time hospice use has grown to encompass the huge number of patients in terminal stages of dementia whereas prior to that time, hospice care was used mostly by a much smaller number of patients with terminal cancer who had a very short time left to live.[2]

True, Alzheimer's disease is technically terminal in that there is no cure, but like other technically terminal illnesses (emphysema and congestive heart failure, for example) persons with Alzheimer's disease might live many months or even years while on hospice. Obviously, with the expansion of hospice services to "chronic and incurable" illnesses such as Alzheimer's, the number of people who qualify for hospice services has increased dramatically, as has the duration of time they can remain on hospice.

Because of the proliferation of hospice providers, hospice is accessible to almost everyone, and while hospice is a wonderful option for those suffering from terminal illness, and is most often used appropriately, we have seen an alarming trend among dementia care facilities to inappropriately refer residents with dementia into hospice programs for reasons other than the terminal nature of the disease. The facilities are sometimes highly motivated by the chance to be relieved of many of their caregiving duties by the hospice service, as shown in the following example.

Effie: At Death's Door?

Effie was a 94-year-old devout Catholic woman who had resided in assisted living in a senior community for seven years. Her daughter (herself in her 70's, and with her own health concerns) provided unflagging support of Effie, visited every day, communicated with physicians, and took Effie to doctors' appointments. Over time, Effie became depressed, developed dementia, and also began having problems with chronic shoulder pain from a torn rotator cuff, but was in generally good physical shape. She was ambulatory with a walker, but needed help dressing and toileting. At this point, Effie moved into the skilled nursing section of the community.

After Effie's move the nursing staff reported that Effie was irritable, and would sometimes yell at and even strike the caregivers. A psychiatrist was working with Effie, the facility, and the family to help resolve the behavioral issues, but because the behavior was linked to pain and because impacting Effie's behavior would require coordinated actions among all the caregivers, changes were slow. One day, out of the blue, Effie's daughter received a call from the social worker with an ultimatum from the facility: either put Effie on hospice, or find another home for Effie. Effie's daughter questioned the social worker further, and was told that since Effie had pain, perhaps the pain was causing her behavioral outbursts, and so the facility wanted to "try" hospice for "a couple of weeks" to see if hospice could resolve the pain. Never had Effie been referred to a pain specialist. Never had Effie's daughter been invited to a care plan meeting to discuss the behavioral problems. Never had Effie been diagnosed with a terminal condition. Somehow, the facility thought that by calling in the psychiatrist, they had adequately addressed Effie's needs, and since the psychiatrist had "failed" to change Effie's behavior (as if the psychiatrist were a substitute for appropriate training in dementia and pain management), there was no other solution than hospice. Effie's daughter reluctantly consented to hospice, and when the psychiatrist questioned the "terminal" nature of Effie's condition, said that she "didn't know (she) had a choice."

This scene is played out with many different variations across the country every day. The particulars are different, but similar tactics of manipulation, threats, or persuasion are used by some facilities to move reluctant families toward hospice. This is due to a number of factors including the facility staff's lack of understanding of the regulations for hospice, and the perception that hospice can be used to provide solutions to problems that the facility cannot handle. This scenario also highlights what can happen when "hospice" care is substituted improperly for palliative care. Clearly, Effie's daughter realized that Effie could not be cured of her dementia, but there was no reason to think that her mother was dying. The suggestion to use hospice seemed to Effie's daughter as if the facility wanted to hasten Effie's death.

APPROPRIATE HOSPICE CARE

In order to understand the context in which hospice care is appropriate, we should look at how hospice payment is structured. Medicare pays for hospice services for certain Medicare beneficiaries. Americans over the age of 65 are the largest group of Medicare beneficiaries. Hospice is paid a *per diem* rate for care, excluding around-the-clock nursing care. The *per diem* rate is the same whether many services are used or few. According to the National Senior Citizens Law Center:

> Medicare rules allow payment for hospice care only if a doctor has certified that the patient is expected to die within six months. If the patient in fact does not die within the six months, hospice care nonetheless can be continued **indefinitely**, as long as the doctor continues to certify that the resident

is expected to die within the following six months. (Author emphasis added) [3]

Note that the qualifying condition (i.e. terminal condition) is subject to physician re-certification, which allows some patients to remain on hospice far longer than six months.

Determining Medicare payment for hospice in the case of Alzheimer's or other dementia is more difficult than for other illnesses because, although Alzheimer's is technically a terminal condition, sometimes a person lives for 10 or 15 years with the disease. In addition, Alzheimer's disease is not the direct cause of death, but kills because of the effects the disease ultimately has on other organ systems. For example, persons with Alzheimer's are particularly susceptible to pneumonia because the swallowing reflex is destroyed over time by death of the neurons that control this function. People who have difficulty swallowing often inhale food or saliva into their lungs and develop "aspiration pneumonia." For these reasons, estimating the life expectancy of a patient with Alzheimer's can be difficult, so hospice companies use various debility scales to categorize functional level and predict prognosis for hospice eligibility under Medicare. The Reisberg Functional Assessment Staging (FAST) Scale is the most commonly used. [4] You might have heard people talk about what "stage" of Alzheimer's a person is in. Well, that staging comes from the FAST Scale and others like it. There are seven stages to the FAST Scale, and a person at stage 7 is likely to be advanced enough in the disease process to qualify for a prognosis of death within six months. Items assessed in the FAST Scale include degree of memory loss (i.e. losing items, forgetting events, not recognizing people), ability to toilet independently, ability to dress independently, eat independently and finally even sit up or hold up one's head. It is important to realize that the FAST Scale only takes into account the debility associated with Alzheimer's disease. This is why a person with Alzheimer's can have a low FAST Scale score, but still be eligible for hospice because of other, co-morbid diseases such as cardiovascular disease. The evaluation of co-morbid and secondary conditions is complex, so you should confer with the hospice provider of your choice for more information.

What hospice services are covered by Medicare? Medicare does not pay for room costs associated with assisted living, but Medicare will pay for hospice services within assisted living facilities. There are some restrictions, though. According to the National Senior Citizens Law Center:

> Hospice care should not replace anything that a facility otherwise is obligated to do. Instead, hospice services should supplement and improve upon the facility-provided services. [3]

We have sometimes seen hospice care used to replace the care the facility is required by law to provide. For example, care staff employed by the assisted living community might have been giving medication to a patient, helping him with meals, dressing, and bathing long before the resident begins receiving hospice care, but under hospice, there are additional caregivers sent to take over some of those duties. Families call hospice staff rather than assisted living nurses when they have questions. Grief counseling provided by pastoral or social work staff from hospice takes the place of services that the assisted living community can provide through referrals to psychologists and other counselors. Once hospice care is initiated, services formerly provided by the assisted living staff are provided by hospice so that in fact, hospice may be duplicating services provided by the assisted living. "Extra" nursing care by hospice means that there is, in reality, less nursing care that the patient or family is requesting from the assisted living staff.

In reality, it's almost impossible to completely partition care given by hospice from that given by the assisted living staff. However, this duplication of services provides its own incentive for hospice referral. Since assisted living facilities usually do not lower their rates even though some (often many) of their tasks are being performed by hospice, the resident is, in essence, paying twice but receiving services only once. (Actually, the resident is paying once and the public is making duplicate payments since Medicare is supported through tax dollars). Medicare is also subsidizing assisted living care provided to non-hospice residents since the hospice services provided to some patients allow assisted living staff to have more time to spend with non-hospice residents.

So, looking at the regulations, while Effie's hospice referral was legal, it was not necessarily appropriate. Because of their ignorance about dementia and appropriate pain control the staff at Effie's community were improperly attributing Effie's symptoms to an end-stage process, rather than seeing them as reversible, and following through with appropriate care.

How Do Hospice Companies Work?

When hospice was first introduced, it was never meant to be a form of long-term care or to substitute for long-term care. We have indicated earlier in this book that in some ways, assisted living has become the "new nursing home." More residents are remaining in assisted living while receiving hospice services rather than transitioning to nursing facilities. This makes sense, since hospice care can be provided in the home, and for most assisted living residents, the assisted living community is, in fact, home, so there really is no reason to transition from assisted living to a nursing home. If you have ever been part of a move into or out of assisted living, you can understand that avoiding that painful process is very attractive to residents and their families, as well as being desirable to the assisted living facility itself.

Studies show that even though there was a higher prevalence of residents with moderate to advanced dementia in nursing homes than in assisted living or residential care communities, residents in assisted living and residential care communities received end-of-life or hospice care almost twice as often as their nursing home counterparts. (5,6,7) It is unclear whether nursing home residents with dementia receive end-of-life care by the nursing facilities themselves without hospice assistance, or whether these patients are hospitalized at the end of life. Indeed, there is specialized nursing care already in place within nursing homes, so that nursing homes are able to care for medical problems that assisted living cannot. This is because nursing staff in assisted living is limited, as you recall from earlier in this book. Clearly then, assisted living offers a rich source of potential patients for the hospice industry.

There are hospice providers that are "for profit" and others that are "non-profit." The four largest for-profit hospice companies are Vitas®, Odyssey®, HCR ManorCare®, and VistaCare®. All four are publicly-traded companies, meaning that they are beholden to stockholders who expect dividends, or a return on investment. Of the four, Vitas® is the largest. Founded by a minister and a nurse in 1978, Vitas® now operates in eight states: California, Florida, Illinois, New Jersey, Ohio, Pennsylvania, Texas and Wisconsin. Its nearly 6,000 employees provide care for patients in its own inpatient hospice units, or in homes, nursing homes, assisted living facilities, and hospitals. No longer owned by the founders, Vitas® is now owned by Chemed Corporation—the parent company of Roto Rooter®—who paid over $406 million dollars for the company. [8]

The tempting reaction to the inherent distaste many of us feel for what seems to be death profiteering is to declare that hospice should be "non-profit." Let's look at that logically for a moment. First, it is important to know that "non-profit" is really just a classification used by the Internal Revenue Service to determine tax status and, in and of itself, does not confer any moral superiority or inherent philanthropy. Indeed, non-profit entities can operate businesses that charge for services. At the very least, non-profits have boards of directors to keep happy (some directors receive payment for their board service) and employee salaries to pay. Even non-profit companies can pay high salaries to the executives or pay bonuses from the profits.

So, even a "non-profit" corporation has a real incentive to maximize the bottom line, which means taking in more money than it spends in order to keep services available to its customers. Non-profit hospices expend a considerable amount of time and effort soliciting donations. A little-known fact is that for-profit hospices can receive charitable donations as well, but they cannot actually solicit such donations. Have you had a friend or relative who died, and the family requests that, instead of flowers, donations to a hospice company be made?

You may not have known whether the company was for-profit or non-profit at the time.

Non-profit hospice providers still account for about two-thirds of the hospice care provided nationally, but comparison of publicly traded hospices versus their non-profit counterparts is interesting. For example, one study has found that "for-profit hospices compared to non-profit hospices serve a higher percentage of persons with non-cancer diagnoses, residents of long-term care, and persons with government insurance."[9] The real question, though, is not the tax status of a hospice, but whether a hospice's bottom line actually influences the quality of care it provides. Studies seem to indicate that non-profit hospices provide more highly trained staff and more services, and that families are more satisfied with the care their loved ones receive compared to for-profit hospices. [9]

A very recent trend that may become more prevalent is for a long-term care community to provide its own hospice service. Thus, a separate agency would not be contracted to provide services, but the community would hire its own hospice staff to provide services within its own facility. This begs the question: Will a community that provides its own hospice program save the patient money, or will it further blur the line between care by the facility and care by hospice? It remains to be seen.

MARKETING DEATH

The marketing of hospice to long-term care facilities has been insidious. Wait, you say—marketing hospice? Yes. Is marketing bad? Not at all. In fact, marketing is a way that the dying and their families can receive information— not about the existence of hospice, but about the various options available to them. While marketing can have a legitimate place in hospice provision, the trouble begins when the marketer and the consumer lose sight of potential conflicts of interest. Remember, marketing is employed with a very clear goal in mind—to increase referrals.

Many hospice providers employ full-time marketing personnel. There are websites where you can find helpful marketing ideas for hospice. Halloween marketing, cookie marketing—you name it. One company describes how, when a hospice patient dies, the company sends information to that patient's doctor describing what hospice services were given to the patient, who was present at death, and a handwritten note to thank the physician for the referral. Many tactics and terms are used to formalize the marketing processes that companies use. Designating a key administrator in the hospice company to establish relationships with individual physicians or practice groups in order to increase dependable referrals from those physicians, or writing letters to the editor of the local newspaper to enhance the reputation of hospice are two strategies. Pens with hospice logos appear at the nursing station at the assisted living community. Then direct care workers employed by the residential community begin wearing identification badge holders emblazoned with the name of one or another hospice. Sometimes, staff will receive a box of donuts or candy as a "thank you" gift from a hospice provider, and sometimes, lunch is provided.

What if a nurse recommends a hospice simply because he happens to have a hospice-supplied pen with the referral number in his hand at the time? What if that nurse really prefers the care given by Hospice A, but he would feel embarrassed if Hospice B came with their usual Friday lunch and found that he had referred a patient somewhere else? We are all vulnerable to the powerful force of being liked, and we all tend to avoid the more powerful force of being shunned. These forces are definitely at play in any face-to-face marketing such as that which happens when hospice providers market to facilities.

Hospice marketers advise assisted living communities to begin discussions about end-of-life issues when the resident first enters the facility. Mandatory end-of-life "inservices" have begun appearing more and more often— usually led by a member of a local hospice team. Assisted living communities may also contract with specific hospice providers to provide services exclusive to their residents.

So, as you can see, there is a blurring of roles in hospice marketing. The marketing drives a conflict of interest in which assisted living employees are potentially biased in the information they provide to vulnerable residents and their families. We know for a fact that assisted living employees (a) are rarely aware of the regulations affecting hospice, and (b) do not receive ethics training regarding the conflicts of interest inherent in the marketing relationships. Far from being intentionally unethical, uneducated administrators and caregivers may see hospice as the most likely way to get extra help for providing resident care in a time of understaffing.

WHAT CAN YOU DO?

So, we have seen that, although hospice has a legitimate place in assisted living, especially in dementia care, there are many pitfalls for residents and their families. Like Effie's daughter in the story at the start of this chapter, many families feel pressured, unknowledgeable, and even trapped when hospice is presented as an option. The first thing families can do is to understand the difference between end-of-life palliative care (which does not need to be provided by a specialized hospice model) and hospice care, which is designed to help the patient and family transition through the dying process. The Texas Non-profit Hospice Alliance suggests asking the following questions of any hospice provider:

- How long have you been providing hospice services in our community?
- What is your ratio of staff to patients?
- Do you have hospice-certified nurses?
- What out-of-pocket expenses are there for medications, equipment, and supplies?
- What medications are not provided?
- What kinds of post-death support do you provide for the family?
- How often will your staff make personal visits?
- What is the quickest way to reach you, and what is your response time?
- What sets you apart from other local hospice providers?
- Are you a non-profit organization?
- Why do you do this work? [10]

In addition to these questions, we suggest that you:

1) Be certain you know why hospice care is being recommended. If it is for convenience or for a behavior problem, work with the staff to determine other options. Don't accept strong-arm tactics, veiled threats, or warnings that without hospice your loved one will not get proper care or pain control.

2) Ask your physician what hospice can provide that he or she can't. Ask whether your personal physician or the hospice physician will ultimately decide

issues of care and medication. Ask your physician if he or she is willing to provide palliative care and if he/she understands the difference between palliative and hospice care.

3) Ask the assisted living residence what their policy is on duplication of services between hospice and facility staff. Ask if the cost of assisted living will change and how it will change if hospice provides services.

4) Ask the hospice what the policy is about intravenous hydration for comfort, treatment of conditions such as fractures, pneumonia, or heart failure.

5) Ask what their training in dementia care is. Can they discern the reasons for agitation in patients with dementia?

6) Ask for references from other families, and go online and research the hospice agency.

Above all, don't be intimidated from asking tough questions both before and during the time you work with hospice. Don't assume that the hospice staff are the experts and your questions are without merit. As you would with all other products and services, be an educated consumer.

But know this: If the staff taking care of your family member is not adequately or appropriately trained, there is a high likelihood that behavior changes will be interpreted as simply the progression of the disease, and the "end-of-life" discussion may begin too soon or unnecessarily.

REFERENCES

1. World Health Organization Definition of Palliative Care. Accessed at: www.who.int/cancer/palliative/definition/en/

2. Campbell DE, Lynn J, Louis TA, Shugarman LR; Medicare Program Expenditures Associated with Hospice Use. *Annals of Internal Medicine*, 2004: 140:4, pp. 269-277

3. National Senior Citizens Law Center: Paying for Assisted Living http://www.nsclc.org/consumer/paying-for-assisted-living/?searchterm=hospice

4. Reisberg B. Functional assessment staging. *Psychopharmacol Bull.* 1988;24(4):653-9

5. Magaziner J, German P, Zimmerman SI, Hebel JR, Burton L, Gruber-Baldini AL, May C, Kittner S. The prevalence of dementia in a statewide sample of new nursing home admissions aged 65 and older: diagnosis by expert panel. Epidemiology of Dementia in Nursing Homes Research Group. *Gerontologist.* 2000 Dec;40(6):663-72

6. Hawes C, Phillips CD, Rose M, et al. A National Survey of Assisted Living Facilities, *Gerontologist,* 43(6):875-882

7. Sloane PD, Zimmerman S, Hanson L, et al. End-of-life care in assisted living and related residential care settings: Comparison with nursing homes. *J Am Geriatr Soc.*2003;51:1587-1594

8. Chemed Corp.: Major Player in Hospice and Plumbing. February26,2007www.seekingalpha.com/article/28067-chemed-corp-player-in-hospice-and-plumbing.

9. McCue MJ, Thompson JM, Operational and Financial Performance of publicly traded hospice companies *J Palliative Med* 2005 Dec; 8(6): 1196-206

10. Texas Non-Profit Hospice Alliance. Accessed at: http://www.tnpha.org/

CHAPTER SIX
WHY IS THIS SO DIFFICULT?

Ultimately, most families face the same question: "How will I know when it's time to place my family member in long-term care?" The answer is not simple. Research shows there are a number of reasons why people with dementia are placed in facilities, but the main reason is the burden that the caregiver perceives. [1] At what point does the burden take precedence over all else? That's difficult, too. We have repeatedly heard caregivers who have thought about placement and have determined what, for them, would "definitely" result in the decision to place a loved one. Examples of such "definite" triggers include things such as, "Well, when I have to change my wife's (husband's, father's, mother's) diaper, then I will know it will be time to put her in a facility" or "if he starts wandering, then I'll know he's not safe to stay at home anymore." Then, before they realize it, the family is changing diapers, or they have hired full-time help to prevent the wandering, but no one seems to think it is such a burden after all, so they keep their loved one at home.

Who is to say how much "burden" is enough to make it acceptable to place your parent or spouse or sibling in a facility for more care? The ability to tolerate ever-escalating care demands because placement has such bad connotations seems to be a key to caregiver stress. Family squabbles and even family legal battles are fought over appropriate care, but often, the real issues are guilt, fear, and betrayal.

The truth is, caregiver burden is a concept that everyone can identify with, but the specific idea of what constitutes "burden" is different for everyone. What about the person with dementia who is compliant with care but who has to wear diapers, needs to be fed, and has to be bathed? Is that person less, or more, of a burden than the person who fights and hits whenever personal care is attempted, but is otherwise good natured, eats well, and can hold a conversation?

To make things even more complicated, research also reveals that placement of a loved one in a facility really does not reduce the sense of caregiver burden.[2] It seems as if one set of worries is traded for another, whether real or anticipated. So, if you think that placing your relative in a facility will solve all the problems and eliminate stress, that may not be the case—at least not entirely.

MARKETING TACTICS

So now that your family member's care has crossed your personal "burden limit" or you need to take action to make them safe as soon as possible, or other issues have arisen that require intervention, your first education will be in marketing. That the long-term care industry markets its products and services should come as no surprise. Marketing is a primary concern for both for-profit and non-profit facilities. Without marketing, how will people know that services are available? Advertising and marketing in any industry or service area is designed to have an emotional impact on consumers. As you will learn in this chapter, the industry might not make intentional efforts to make too many promises or to misrepresent the level of care they can provide, but the fact is that the promotion of elder services hits all the emotional buttons associated with aging and elder care. Those emotional buttons include guilt, fear, and a myriad of personal inadequacies that people bring to the table. Marketing necessarily capitalizes on the power of these emotions to influence our decisions. When you couple such emotional hotspots with the fact that very few of us make it to adulthood without carrying over some issues from childhood, the situation in which an adult child has to cope with the necessity of caring for a debilitated parent is a set-up for making emotional rather than rational decisions.

So what do you do when you have to think about finding a secure dementia unit for a father who was a world traveler and ran his own successful multi-million dollar business? Or when you are in the heartbreaking position in which you must provide full-time care for a mother who always cared for you? Well, you might start by looking at websites and brochures where you will find words such as "familiarity," "trust," "respect," "commitment," and "protect" littered throughout the paragraphs. You will frequently see descriptions such as "homelike setting," "innovative approach to caring," "personalized surroundings," "trained staff available 24 hours a day," "a safe haven," "ongoing support," "quality assurance," " open communication," "well-trained staff," "customized services," or "individualized service plan."

You can see how such general comments could lead you—intentionally or not—to inaccurate assumptions about staff's expertise in dementia. In your state of crisis, with emotional buttons primed and pushed, you and your loved one will pay attention to the carefully placed key words "safe," "trust," "secure," "compassionate," "protects," "valued and loved," "trained, professional staff," and "around the clock." As was the marketing intention, you experience a level of cautious relief, easing the transition to the new lifestyle, because you (and most other consumers) translate these words through the filter of your own emotional state. Here are some examples:

"Well-trained staff"

The staff is so much more knowledgeable than I am, so I can trust them to take care of Mom and safely manage any crisis that arises.

"A safe haven for seniors"

I can trust these people to watch out for Dad so he will feel at home and won't be in any danger anymore. Some of the burden will be lifted off of me and he'll even be better off.

"Family involvement"

I will continue to be a part of Mom's life, rather than just "placing" her and paying the bills. Also, they must be trustworthy, or else they wouldn't want families involved.

"Assistance with medications"

I won't have to worry about Dad's health because I can trust the staff to see that he won't miss his medications, and his medications will be given correctly. I was really unsure about my ability to do that properly anyway.

"Open communication"

I can trust the facility to tell me what's going on with Mom, and I can speak my mind without fear of rebuke or judgment. Information won't be hidden.

Messages such as the ones above reach out in an extraordinarily powerful way to desperate families in need of solutions in their time of crisis. However, as comforting as these messages are for families that are hurting, families have repeatedly told us that what they really need is a way to **reliably** compare the services offered by various facilities. Unfortunately, the chance of obtaining the specific details necessary to make an accurate comparison between facilities is unlikely.

Not only is the information scattered and often of poor quality, but facilities literally refuse to provide needed information. For example, in 2005, *Consumer Reports* magazine requested information from 35 facilities owned by the top ten corporate providers of assisted living services. [3] Only four facilities reported information about "staff training," and four provided information about "who administers medications." Note that the majority of facilities didn't simply provide poor information, they provided no information at all on the vital questions about training and medication administration. If these data are poorly accessible to a major consumer publication like *Consumer Reports*, how much more difficult is it for individual consumers?

Even if individual facilities are cooperative and helpful in providing information to inquiring families, an enormous amount of time and energy is required to catalogue the information so that a consumer can compare apples to apples. Besides, in their emotional distress most consumers do not ask nuts-and-bolts questions about operational practices such as specific training and staff levels, or what particular professional level is required of the person who is taking care of the resident. Certainly, it is a rare assisted living facility that would address such questions in their marketing materials. Often, consumers are looking for an assisted living facility under time pressure (i.e., the "burden limit"), because, for instance, there is either a crisis situation or the prospective resident needs extensive assistance from family members whose time is limited.

All of the problems we described above become even trickier if you are trying to find a residence for a loved one in another state. You may presuppose that the training and facility guidelines are the same as the state in which you live. However, if you recall the discussion in Chapter 3 about the variety in quality or even presence of training requirements from state to state, you will see that any difficulties inherent in facility comparison are only compounded by the variety of state requirements, definitions, and regulations. When looking for facilities in another state, it may be even more likely that a family's decisions are based on faulty assumptions and false hopes.

What can you do? Well, first, see if state survey information is available for the facilities you are considering. By federal law, individual states conduct "inspections of each nursing home that participates in Medicare and/or Medicaid on average about once a year." [4] This is not true for assisted living, but some nursing homes have sections of the facility that provide specialized dementia care. Each facility subject to the state inspection process is required by law to make the latest state inspection report available for examination in a place readily accessible to residents and, therefore, families.

Another option is to attend an Alzheimer's or dementia support group and ask the other group members about their actual experiences with various facilities. Ask your (or your loved one's) physician where they would place a loved one. Attempt to do assisted living comparisons on the Internet. Ask the assisted living administrator for specific training policies and procedures for the various facilities in writing and save the information in a binder to compare. Likewise, ask for staffing levels—both during the day and at night.

THE PERSONAL TOUCH

It is no secret that people make many purchases based on emotions rather than reason. Marketing experts in assisted living know that families and prospective residents are usually in a crisis or near-crisis when they walk through the doors of the facility. They take great care to ensure that your first encounter with facility staff is a positive one. There is absolutely nothing wrong with that, but keep in mind that the person with whom you speak on your first visit to a facility may not be a health care professional. The person is rarely identified as "marketing" staff, but may have a title like "Community Outreach" or "Intake Coordinator." Such titles further blur the line between knowledgeable health care provider and effective sales person. The trust you have in that person's credibility is based at least in part on their title. Even though they might be very trustworthy and dedicated, that person's job is to sell the services of the facility to consumers.

Once a consumer is in the facility, external appearances rise to a place of huge importance. Why is it that assisted living facilities seem to place more emphasis on external appearances than staff development or resident care when dealing with prospective clients? There are probably a lot of complex reasons, including genuine pride in beautifully landscaped outdoor areas and tasteful décor, but facility administrators have also admitted to us that the décor and architecture are mainly to help families and friends assuage their guilt about placing a loved one in a long-term care facility. By making the consumer feel special while they visit a facility, the marketing team starts to sell abstract ideas like "trust" and "homelike" rather than facilitating rational decisions based on measurable information. The goal is to engage the consumer with good social skills, a focus on positives, and the right "attitude." After all, when families are in crisis, a reassuring smile goes a long way. Again, this is not to say that décor, cleanliness, and friendliness are not extremely important, but we want to warn you not to overlook operational nuts and bolts such as training, staffing, and policies.

What about brochures? Although facilities typically supply families with a great deal of written information (albeit vague) most consumers subconsciously rely on what they are told verbally by managers and administrators. This, of course, is human nature. On an instinctive level, most of us trust the people with whom we have developed a relationship more than we trust written material. Later, when consumers might be comparing various brochures to make decisions, the memory of a warm relationship often trumps a slick brochure that looks much like all of the others.

What does assisted living really sell? To answer that question, we must first recognize that the commodity sold by assisted living and the services sought by consumers might be different. When families ask us as experts in dementia and elder care to recommend options for care for their loved one with dementia, they do not ask which facility has the best lobby furniture, the best food, or even the friendliest staff. They ask us for recommendations of places that provide safety, individualized activities, readily available assistance for any need, and well-trained staff that can manage their loved one's dementia-related behaviors. So, going back to our original question – what does assisted living really sell? Expertise? Compassionate care? Safety? Wellness? Maybe all of those, but what is really for sale is TRUST. Think back on the language used in the marketing materials discussed earlier in this chapter. They certainly seem to be selling lots of things, but the underlying concept of each of those comments is TRUST.

So the stage is set. The facility has successfully engendered trust in a prospective client, and with that trust comes expectation. Families and residents have many expectations, including any combination or all of the following: safety, better health, better mood, improved behavior, weight gain, more social outings, less arguing, less fear, more affection, or better grooming. Because families and residents are in crisis, and they need to believe they have chosen the "right" facility for a loved one, the expectations are high and the consequences of misplaced trust can be tragic.

One could argue that trust is being sold in any sales transaction—not just assisted living. For example, we trust that the food we buy will be fresh; we trust that the car we buy will run. While this is certainly true, the level of trust required to turn over the care of a loved one—a child or an elder—is much higher and has a greater emotional component. If our food is not fresh, we complain and move on. When the car breaks down as we are driving off the lot, we return it under the Lemon Law. But when our trust in the care of a loved one is betrayed, can we simply complain and move on or "take it back?" Not really, because moving into an assisted living facility is a total disruption of a person's lifestyle and habits. It is a highly stressful event for both the prospective resident and the family. Feeling able to trust the facility assuages some of the guilt, but if that trust is betrayed, families feel guilty about having placed trust in "strangers" in the first place. Of course, this is compounded when the elder bitterly opposed the move in the first place. Depending on the severity of the "betrayal," consumer guilt turns to anger, which turns to thoughts of lawsuits and vengeance.

Although it is difficult to escape the emotional snares inherent in family decisions such as long-term care, it is very important to try to separate actual facts and figures from your emotional reaction to a facility. As we have emphasized before, gather all of the objective data possible. Talk to residents and, if possible, former residents and their families. Also, go to the facility at night, on weekends, and during change of shift. Hire an attorney or paralegal to research the lawsuit history on a particular facility if possible.

AFTER THE MOVE

If things go badly after having moved into a facility, "buyer's remorse" takes on a whole new meaning. The family or the resident may begin to wonder: Did I make a mistake? Was I fooled into thinking this was a good place? Was I rushed to make a decision without enough information? To foil those doubts, consumers often try to rationalize the failings of the facility. For instance, one might say, "Aides cannot be expected to know very much, because they are so poorly paid," or "I should be more involved in order to make sure things don't go wrong," or "There have been so many different managers that they just can't keep up." Unfortunately, good money is paid for high levels of care, but many deficiencies in care are rationalized and accepted by both providers and families. The problem with this is that these beliefs become obstacles to improving care in a facility, and if poor care continues while residents or families feel powerless, they also feel increasingly resentful which further impedes any communication that might help resolve the problems. Let's look at some faulty beliefs as well as legitimate fears that we have seen become obstacles to better care.

Belief #1: <u>If I or my loved one is a compliant, friendly resident, then the staff will provide better care and lots more attention.</u> While there are no scientific studies about this issue, we can tell you from our experience with facilities that this is a faulty belief. What really happens is the resident who yells, hits, is found crying, wanders, or argues with staff is the resident who receives lots of attention (even though not all positive), more family communication by staff (to report all the behaviors and problems), more contacts with the physician, and more consults from mental health care providers (to help determine why the resident is behaving in a certain way or to give medications to solve the behavior problems). It is the quiet, friendly resident that is left alone, because he or she seems fairly self-sufficient and seems obedient.

Obviously, we are not advocating that residents and families should cause problems to get attention, but residents and families should make needs known to the appropriate staff members—going up the management chain if necessary. It is critically important once you have made needs known that you request an action plan and accountability. In most states, a formal care plan is required to be developed for each resident, and you have the right to be involved in that care plan development— whether you are the resident or the family. Do it. In our years of experience with residents of all different kinds of long-term care facilities, we have seen that only about

5% of residents or families takes advantage of care plan participation. Possibly, we are seeing a skewed population of residents who are not involved in care planning, but remember, the patients we see are often the ones with the most problems. Either way—whether there are problems or you want to avoid problems, skipping the care planning is not a good idea.

Belief #2: If I am friendly and compliant, my loved one will get better care. Again, there are no scientific studies, but our experience with families and facilities tells us otherwise. Yes, the staff are friendly to compliant residents and families and are glad to see them, but it is most likely because the staff don't perceive compliant consumers as being demanding. What is considered "too demanding?" Sadly, we have seen that even ongoing questions and accountability are considered "too demanding" by some staff. Too often staff becomes defensive if questions are asked, even if those questions are genuine and not posed in a confrontational way. Even so, it is important to continue to participate in care plans, keep an open line of communication with caregivers, social workers, and administrators and attend family or resident council meetings. Of course, it goes without saying that threats, bribes, coercion or temper tantrums do not constitute "open" lines of communication. (Unfortunately, we have seen families and residents do all of these things.) Even when emotions are high, it is important to be respectful and factual. Finally, do not forget to maintain communication with the physician overseeing care. Often, events transpire without the doctors' even being aware. Sadly, sometimes this is because the doctor isn't involved enough, but sometimes no one has thought to inform the doctor.

Belief #3: <u>If I complain or make a fuss, the staff will take it out on my loved one</u>. This is the greatest fear of all. To leave the facility after having had disagreements about care, fearing what the night may hold for your parent, spouse, or friend is horrifying. Unfortunately, we are sad to say that there is evidence that retribution happens. However, we are certain that if training and family-resident-staff communication were improved, not only would families' fear of retribution be diminished, but also staff would feel less frustrated and angry. Remember that staff training has multiple benefits besides better care, and among them is an increased sense of staff professionalism and confidence in appropriate care. In other words, staff who are treated with the dignity of corporate investment in education have been proven to be more compassionate and professional in their care of elders. For all these reasons, families would be more comfortable in airing concerns.

If you are in a situation where you are concerned about retribution, there are a few things you can do. Stay with your loved one, or hire a sitter. Document any threats and any changes in appearance, nutrition, or demeanor of your loved one. If you think there has been retribution, report it to the state regulatory agency. You may indeed need to move your loved one to another facility.

Belief #4: <u>If I complain, they will kick us out</u>. While retribution is a big fear for families, being "evicted" from the facility is a close second. Recall how accommodating the staff can be when you are in the process of making the decision to use the facility. Now all of a sudden they are unable to do the very things they assured you were routine. This situation is similar to the one above where families are concerned that "difficult" resident behavior might lead to eviction, but in this case the sense is that if the family is not cooperative or asks too many questions, the resident will need to find another place to live.

If this happens to you, first, make sure you know the facility's stated policies on eviction. Next, talk to the physician caring for your loved one. If there is a sympathetic nurse, aide, or social worker, enlist his or her help in rectifying the situation. As we emphasized above, make sure you attend the care plan meetings (if your facility has them) so that you are alerted to any potential bases the facility might have for eviction. Finally, listen respectfully to the concerns the facility has. They really might be feeling threatened not so much by your involvement as by your attitude. Likewise, they might honestly be telling you that, despite their best efforts, they are unable to provide your loved one with the care he or she needs. Not that this is necessarily right, especially if they promised you more when you were touring the facility. However, wouldn't you rather have your loved one in a safe place that is qualified to care for him or her appropriately than to "win" and keep getting inadequate care—even if you don't have to move?

Belief #5: <u>If my loved one causes too much work for the staff, we will be asked to find another facility</u>. Because of the often realistic fear of retributive or frivolous lawsuits, staff can seem evasive or even secretive when you ask questions about changes in behavior or odd accusations. If your loved one has increasing care needs or has behavior changes, you will likely be surprised that, despite your friendly manner or non-complaining attitude, the manager might ask that you remove your "difficult" loved one from the facility. Let's look at an example of this.

Mr. Johnson: Good Samaritan or Let No Good Deed Go Unpunished?

Mr. Johnson had just moved into an assisted living community. At first, he seemed to be adjusting well. Although he had significant memory problems and some episodes of confusion and sometimes had difficulty finding his way to his room, his social skills seemed appropriate.

Despite this auspicious beginning, after he had been at the facility for several days, Mr. Johnson became irritating to some of the other residents. As people in wheelchairs made their way to the dining room, some would stop to visit with each other or to look out the window. When he saw someone whose wheelchair was stopped, Mr. Johnson would immediately go up behind them and begin pushing the wheelchairs toward the dining room. Such sudden, unexpected movement would startle the residents, especially because they could not see who was behind them. His behavior was met with fear and anger by these other residents. Some of them would start to scream and flail their arms, while others would call out, "Who are you? What are you doing?" Mr. Johnson would then become confused about their reaction and would usually try to lower their flailing arms, although sometimes he would curse at them and walk away.

The director of the facility contacted Mr. Johnson's doctor and told him that Mr. Johnson had become agitated and was "assaulting" the residents. The staff at the facility thought Mr. Johnson needed medication or perhaps needed to move to a secured dementia care unit. The doctor provided a prescription for a strong tranquilizer to be used "as needed." The staff would *attempt to administer the medication to Mr. Johnson when they observed him in an agitated state, but by that time, he was usually so upset that he would refuse the medicine and curse at the staff.*

Sometimes a staff member would notice that Mr. Johnson was starting to move someone's wheelchair and could successfully intervene by engaging him in a conversation or introducing him to the person in the wheelchair. However, such intervention seldom occurred because usually all the staff members were preparing for meal service and were not monitoring the hallway.

The real problem in situations like the one described above is that people who do not know very much about dementia often interpret the behavior of a person with dementia as intentional and planned, when, in fact, the behavior can be quite impulsive. Someone with Alzheimer's or another form of dementia will respond to a situation "in the moment" rather than take into consideration all the factors involved and the consequences of actions. This inability to sequence, plan and appreciate consequences is a hallmark of Alzheimer's and was true in the case of Mr. Johnson. He saw the person in a wheelchair as someone who had stopped moving. He did not understand that they were socializing or enjoying the view out the window. When he pushed them and they startled, he was unable to understand why they responded in such a way because his brain could not interpret their behavior in the context of the situation. Because of his malfunctioning brain, Mr. Johnson interpreted the other residents' behavior as a threat to him, so he responded in kind. Put another way, his not understanding the situation led to his "mirroring" the other residents' behavior. Mirroring is a common behavior in people with Alzheimer's because their brain impairment causes misinterpretation of what is going on around them.

In this case, the staff recognized that Mr. Johnson was trying to move others' wheelchairs for them, but because the staff did not comprehend why he behaved this way, they could not anticipate his behavior. They simply presumed that he was being intentional and purposeful in his actions, so they assumed that he was "agitated" and was "assaulting" the other residents. They did not understand how the brain of a person with dementia malfunctions and affects behavior. However, regardless of their lack of understanding of dementia-related behavior, they should have realized sooner, based on previous experience that they needed to routinely intervene with him before he tried to push the other residents' wheelchairs.

A simple solution would have been to have an aide always escort him to meals, thereby providing him with the guidance and redirection that he needed. In addition, routinely introducing him to the people in the wheelchairs would have provided Mr. Johnson with an appropriate social interaction. However, because the staff did not understand why such interventions would work, no behavior modification plan was implemented to prevent his problem behavior.

Eventually, the staff's lack of understanding of the nature and cause of behaviors associated with dementia led the facility's management to "recommend" that Mr. Johnson be moved to another facility. Clearly, it was not his dementia that resulted in the move to another facility; rather, it was the staff's inability to manage the symptoms associated with Mr. Johnson' dementia.

Sadly, once a facility decides you or your loved one is no longer "appropriate" to stay there, there is usually little you can do. The best thing to do is to make sure that as soon as problems arise, you take steps to address them and reassure the facility that you are not looking to start a legal battle. If a loved one develops behavioral problems, urge consultation with a psychiatrist or psychologist experienced in dealing with dementia. Often (as you learned earlier in this book) "behavior problems" are really behavior management problems. If your loved one makes accusations against staff members, don't automatically assume he or she is lying or delusional. Check it out. Is the accusatory behavior out of character? Could a loved one with dementia be attempting to tell you something but not have the words to express the problem? Spend more time with him or her quietly observing, so that you have real information with which to counter staff's claims of "problem" behavior. As we discussed in Chapter 2, the media is littered with stories of abuse or exploitation of elders in long-term care facilities. Although we do not believe this is the rule, it does happen, and the perpetrators are often aided by the fact that people often dismiss elders and their concerns. The ugly fact of ageism allows elders to be exploited.

There are really no easy answers. Elder care is complex, and the very nature of aging ensures that as soon as you have one hurdle cleared, there will be another.

REFERENCES

1. Kristine Yaffe, MD; Patrick Fox, PhD; Robert Newcomer, PhD; Laura Sands, PhD; Karla Lindquist, MS; Kyle Dane, BS; Kenneth E. Covinsky, MD,MPH. Patient and Caregiver Characteristics and Nursing Home Placement in Patients With Dementia *JAMA*. 2002;287:2090-2097.

2. Chenier, MC. Review and analysis of caregiver burden and nursing home placement. *Geriatric Nursing* 1997;18(3):121-6.

3. "Assisted Living. How much assistance can you really count on? *Consumer Reports.* July, 2005: 28-33.

4. Medicare information available at: http://www.medicare.gov/Nursing/AboutInspections.asp (accessed 3-29-09).

CHAPTER SEVEN
WHAT YOU CAN DO

After reading much of this book, you may be asking yourself why you would even consider care in a facility at all. You may be thinking, "With all its problems, assisted living and other long-term care options carry too many risks." Instead of avoiding the issues, there are ways that you can manage the whole process and feel more empowered. Instead of feeling helpless at the mercy of so-called experts who assure you they will take care of your loved one, you can feel more confident about directing the care that your loved one receives. You can be a resource and a solution rather than a passive recipient of services you aren't happy with. Really, isn't this the best way to assure quality care for your family member? So what can you do?

EDUCATION

Consumers need to be educated about aging, dementia, legal issues, financial issues, and the dementia care industry. Consider that training yourself is as important as having facility staff who are trained. Consumers need to gain as much understanding as possible in order to communicate better with loved ones and the facility staff. The more you know, the better you can advocate. You are already doing part of this by reading this and other books in order to educate yourself about dementia and issues in long-term care.

In addition to numerous books, there are videos and online resources about dementia. In Appendix A, we have provided some resources that you can use to start your education journey. There is much to learn but do not be put off by the complexity of information or the number of resources. Go at your own speed and interest.

Lectures and seminars are other resources, and they offer you the opportunity to ask questions and communicate. Your local Alzheimer's Association typically has such educational opportunities. In addition, long-term care facilities offer lectures by local or regional experts on many topics. Even though these are marketing efforts aimed at bringing the public in to see a facility, the information provided in the lectures can be quite helpful.

Physicians and other health care providers also can give you helpful information, but you may have to ask specific questions. It is very beneficial for a family member (or members) to accompany the person with dementia to doctors' appointments. Remember, the time you have with the doctor is often limited. Before you go to the doctor with your loved one, write down specific questions you may have. Also write down any changes you have noticed in your loved one's behavior or physical symptoms. If you do not want to reveal information or ask questions in front of your loved one, you can hand written information to the doctor's nurse or fax it to the office beforehand. This way, the doctor will be prepared to give you more information and guidance. Remember, though, to trust your instincts. Sadly, many physicians and nurses are poorly informed about behavioral management in dementia as well as the way that long-term care facilities operate.

ELDER LAW

The specialty of elder law has burgeoned along with the aging population and its many legal concerns, especially considering the changes in estate planning and government subsidies for health care. A consultation with an elder lawyer can help to determine what financial options your loved one has, especially if there is no long-term care insurance policy or if there are family concerns or conflicts. Do not put this off until you are in a crisis situation, when it may be too late for legal intervention to help your loved one. Power of Attorney is not the same as guardianship, and there are limitations on what you can accomplish as you try to intervene to take care of someone. This discussion is beyond the scope of this book, but suffice it to say that you should seek the legal advice you need as soon as you can. The more you know about dementia and the legal implications, the better choices you and your loved one can make. In Appendix A, we list some resources for locating an elder law attorney.

LONG-TERM CARE INSURANCE

Remember Bob and Mary in Chapter 3 of this book? Their story illustrates a couple of the important issues surrounding dementia care in assisted living. Mary faced financial restrictions because of the way long-term care insurance is sometimes structured. Mary didn't—but you can—look for loopholes in long-term care insurance. Remember that although Bob and Mary had long-term care insurance, it would pay only for certain things, requiring Mary to determine how to maximize the help for Bob. The first thing you can do is to be aware that Medicare does not pay for assisted living or for specialized dementia care and only certain states have Medicaid waivers for long-term care in assisted living.

Next, you need to realize that even though long-term care insurance is becoming a prominent factor in financing the care elders need, the insurance providers themselves are not educated about the needs of people with dementia. Consequently, they are not prepared to inform consumers about appropriate options. For example, many insurers talk to their clients about nursing home insurance, and many people believe that they will need only nursing home care, but dementia care is almost always classified as assisted living, so that particular type of care may not be covered in an insurance policy for nursing homes. Many people have had to place loved ones in nursing homes rather than appropriate dementia care assisted living facilities, because of limitations on long-term care insurance. See how it can be tricky?

Once you make sure you have long-term care insurance that will cover dementia care in assisted living, you need to see what the insurance company requires in the way of documentation to trigger payment. Some insurance companies require a formal diagnosis of Alzheimer's and information from the person's doctor indicating the level of care needed in order to justify placement in a facility. The insurance company may also require an evaluation by an independent health care provider in order to evaluate the insured person to justify placement.

Additionally, there may be regularly scheduled evaluations that are required to justify the person's continued stay in the facility. Many elders improve once they become residents of the facility. (This is because the person is often socializing more, taking medications regularly, living in a structured environment, and eating regularly, so health, energy, mood, and basic functions improve.) For some long-term care insurance policies, an improvement in function would then disqualify the person from continuing to reside in an assisted living facility. We know this happens, and it's tragic when an elderly person has to leave a facility in order to deteriorate so that he or she can "prove" to the insurance company the need for continued care in an assisted living.

When considering long-term care insurance, you also need to remember that as Alzheimer's (as well as many other forms of dementia) progresses there will be an increasing need for more services. For instance, you might be able to keep your loved one at home with day care, but later you may need day care and a nighttime caregiver. Then you may need to place that person in specialty dementia care. Then you may need to provide an extra caregiver even in the dementia care facility. Families often do not anticipate the upcoming needs, and at this time in the industry, neither do the insurance companies.

Remember from the initial chapter of this book that dementia is not just Alzheimer's. There can be Parkinson's disease, or dementia from stroke, or heart disease, or damage to the frontal lobe of the brain. Long-term care insurance companies are likely to provide you with statistics about the average length of stay in a nursing home, or the incidence of major illnesses that require special nursing care. However, they may not be able to provide statistical information on the length of stay in a dementia care facility. Regardless, the more you know about dementia and the long-term care industry, the better your questions will be. You will be able to make educated choices about what kind of options you may need from insurance.

COMMUNICATION

Support groups are wonderful sources of information, advice, and assistance. Usually, when people think of support groups, they think of other people's complaining and whining, or they think they will have to bear their souls and weep. Yes, sometimes the viewpoint of others can be uncomfortable, especially those whose family members are at a later stage in the disease process. However, support groups are a great source of ideas, humor, coping skills, and strategies that will carry you forward. Your local Alzheimer's Association has resources, but long-term care facilities may also offer family support groups to the public.

Online discussion groups and message boards are another way to get support without having to leave home or your loved one's presence. For some people it is easier to communicate in the anonymity of an online chat room than face to face. However, sometimes the discussion groups are not moderated, so there can be misinformation and a plethora of somber stories without resolutions. While just expressing your problems and concerns can offer some immediate relief, you may need more help to reduce your stress or to solve a loved one's behavior problem.

There are times when caregivers need individual help. Reluctant to speak in groups, or still holding onto a lot of guilt and shame, some people need one person with whom they can share feelings and thoughts confidentially. Psychologists, social workers, and other professional counselors can be quite helpful to get through tough times. Appendix A provides resources, but also check with your health insurance to see what type of counseling and how much is covered by your policy.

BEST PRACTICES FOR FAMILY COUNCILS

Most long-term care facilities have family councils, either because of state rules or because they want to provide an open forum for communication. The facility's purposes

The Insider's Guide to Dementia Care

for the meetings could be merely to announce some new information, an upcoming event, a solution to a wide-ranging problem, or to introduce new management staff. The family's purpose for the meetings is often quite different.

Families use council meetings as a forum to announce publicly their disappointments or concerns about care practices, in order to bring to the forefront a problem that they have not been able to resolve satisfactorily. Unfortunately, a family council meeting can become a hotbed of angry retorts, accusations, tirades, defensive backpedaling, and ill will.

Family councils work best when a council leader is adept at communicating to all the families without alienating them and when the executive director and nurse manager of the facility are adept at engaging the families and communicating with them outside the public forum. For example, if the administration meets with families about a problem in private or in the context of a resident's care conference, then the problem is less likely to be brought up at the family council meeting and discussed while everyone looks on. During the council meeting, if a family member brings up a problem that has to do with a specific or unique care issue for their loved one, the management staff should make an appointment to discuss it in private.

To assure that your issues are addressed, the best option is to first go to the nurse in charge or another member of the management team. A family's needs will not be met by waiting for a scheduled family council meeting when time is limited and there may be more pressing issues to discuss. So, if you need an issue addressed, seek out management as soon as possible.

Some family council leaders use email to provide

information and an agenda for upcoming meetings. Keeping families "in the loop" lessens the likelihood that they will feel isolated or that they are the only ones with issues. Email is also a way to provide other families with tips and advice on managing care. For instance, if one has found a place to order specialty products for wheelchair-bound or bedridden seniors, then that information could be passed on to other family members who have not had a chance to scour the Internet for products. There are companies starting to offer facilities the chance to have a social network site online that will provide more communication options for staff, residents, and families.

What to Do When Things Go Badly

Facility Management

It is well known that no matter what the industry, be it airlines, restaurants, or long-term care, only one in three people will actually complain about poor service or products. However, those that do not complain will tell an average of 25 people about the poor service and products. Therefore, it behooves the management of the facility to hear you out if you have a complaint. That is really part of management's job, and it is part of your role as family caregiver to express concerns. Remember from previous parts of this book that you may rationalize or dismiss concerns you have, or you may even expect that the issue will not be solved at all. Complaining has negative connotations, and if you would prefer to use the terms "address issues," or "express concerns," or "suggest an idea," feel free. Just remember that whatever you call it, complaining means taking an active role in your loved one's care.

Effective complaining is a skill that takes some practice. In our online course "How Not To Talk," you can practice your approach before you contact the facility manager or nurse manager. The course is a type of role-play. The situation is that you have made a complaint and the nurse at the facility responds to you. You choose your comments from a list of scripted options, the "nurse" character then responds in a scripted way, and subsequently you have a new list of comments from which to choose your answer. In this way, you can "practice" making a complaint, see the facial expression of the other person, and figure out how to respond in the most efficient way. You get feedback on your responses so you can determine the best way (or a better way) to handle the situation. The actual problem situation does not matter as much as the way the complaint is expressed and handled, especially in the context of the nurse character's responses. You can reach it at www. socialanimals.com; click on "caregiver advocacy."

Many people believe that complaining to the aide that takes care of their loved one is the easiest and most immediate way to settle an issue. While this person is a good source of information and support, he or she does not have any authority, especially to direct other caregivers. In addition, aides are most often uninformed about written care plans, new doctor's orders, upcoming appointments, or changes in routines. This means that if you have a complaint or a question, the aide (or resident assistant, as they are sometimes called) may not be able to resolve it. Likewise, the nurse manager can only do so much without the permission of the executive director. In any case, the more you engage management instead of alienating them, the more success you may have in resolving problems.

State Agencies

State agencies that oversee long-term care facilities, even assisted living, have Ombudsman programs. An Ombudsman is a third party who does not work for the facility and is not related to the resident or other family members. He or she is considered to be an objective person with knowledge of state and federal regulations. The Ombudsman investigates complaints made by a resident and/or family members, acts as a spokesperson for the person who made the complaint, and tries to solve the problem or at least offer recommendations for compromise or changes. In some situations it is best to use someone not involved in the problem to mediate and referee. While Ombudsmen have no authority to make changes in regulations or a facility's policies, they can be knowledgeable resources to help reduce the likelihood of continued problems in care. However, there is variability in the effectiveness of Ombudsmen, so the outcome may be a disappointment in some circumstances. Appendix A provides information about how to seek such assistance.

Elected Officials

One resource that is often overlooked by families dealing with long-term care is that of the elected officials of their state. Your state senator or representative will not be able to intervene directly with the facility, but will be able to make inquiries about regulations and regulatory procedures. All you need to do is call the office and talk to an office staff person. Be sure to have details of your situation, in order that the staff person can understand your predicament. Additionally, you should have specific questions, rather than general or vague concerns. This will greatly facilitate the efforts of the office staff helping you.

In addition, it is important to develop and maintain a relationship with your elected representatives because they need input and education about issues that affect their constituents—like you. You see, so much information on so many topics passes across their desks each day that they simply cannot keep up with all of it. Think about it. The state legislators must deal with education, health care, transportation, regulation, environment, insurance, business and many other issues. If you have a relationship with him or her and a bill involving assisted living or elder care comes up, you just might be the "go to" person for that legislator when making a decision about how to vote. Elected officials value the opinions of the people who elect them, and are almost always gracious and willing to talk to you. Again, remember that the legislator will not necessarily intervene except possibly in cases involving regulations or state oversight.

To Sue or Not to Sue

In our litigious society, we often believe that the best results can be achieved with a threatening letter from a lawyer. Sometimes this is true, but in the case of long-term care, this can result in defensive posturing from the facility and alienation of families. One of the reasons that the nursing home industry has difficulty is because it has been bled dry by lawsuits, resulting in enormous increases in liability insurance for the companies that own the facilities or facilities "going bare" (i.e., going without liability insurance). Lawsuits can take years to be resolved, and the legal fees can eat away not only at the resident's savings, but also the savings of family members who are party to the lawsuit.

The legal system is such that the resident can die waiting for resolution of a lawsuit. This is not to say that cases are unworthy of legal attention, but we firmly believe that if a facility's staff is trained to provide appropriate care and the family is educated about dementia, then problems can be met early on and resolved relatively quickly. Training is not a 100% guarantee that there will not be a situation that warrants legal action, but the current sorry state of caregiver training increases the likelihood that problem situations will escalate.

THE CHALLENGE

Consumers need to raise expectations for dementia care and **trust** those expectations. There is no gain when we set our expectations low and make excuses for inadequate care of elders. Think back to Chapter 2 on the example of the three-year-old who is found wandering in the parking lot of the day care center. No one would tolerate low expectations in that situation. Like our children, our elders deserve the best care.

In order to start the process, make observations about the care, make suggestions for improvements or changes, and offer to help solve problems that may seem insurmountable to the administration or the nurses. Learn how to complain and make demands in a way that engages people rather than alienates them. Stop being afraid of retribution. Change your expectation from "This is not so bad, and other aspects of care are okay" to "This is not what I want, so I need to tell them about it so **we** can solve this." You (or your relative) are living in the facility, so you are an expert observer of what happens. If you are a family member, you are the real expert in the care of your loved one. You are the third-party observer whose opinion is, at the very least, equal to others'. Expect that you are a partner in care, not just a helpless recipient.

Evaluate more than the facility exterior when you are making decisions. You may feel comfortable when the décor is pleasing and people are nice, but the real issues can get lost in the process of looking at so many beautiful places. Remember, also, that your loved one's dementia may affect the way the brain processes visual information, so what is pleasant to you may be disturbing or confusing to them.

Of course, asking about details of dementia care training is important. How many hours of dementia care training does the staff receive? How is the training provided: Is it online, in an in-service on payday, in a classroom? Appendix A has a list of resources and further suggestions for questions to ask.

Join advocacy groups and let them know what you are dealing with on a daily basis--both bad and good. Don't use them only as a way to complain, but help them establish the priority of issues. Sometimes advocacy groups focus on an issue, but because their administrators are insulated, they can be unaware there are more important issues that consumers worry about. Advocacy groups can teach you about grassroots initiatives and how to start the process of change on a small local scale. Appendix A lists some advocacy groups that you may contact for more information.

Even if you are a great advocate for yourself or your loved one, you need to recognize that there will continue to be challenges and conflicts. At times it may seem as if the staff in the facility has no interest in doing a better job, or making sure they communicate effectively, or preventing problems. But really, they want to provide the best care for your loved one. Just remember that if more and more families like yours start to change expectations, improve communication, and feel empowered, then the likelihood of real change in long-term care facilities will be realized. It's up to you.

APPENDIX A.

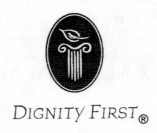

DIGNITY FIRST®

RESOURCES

CONSUMER CHECKLISTS FOR ASSESSING ASSISTED LIVING FACILITIES

Assisted Living Federation of America
1650 King St Ste 602
Alexandria, VA 22314-2747, 703-894-1805.
http://www.alfa.org/files/public/ALFAchecklist.pdf
(Or go to www.alfa.org , click on "Publications and Resources," then click on "Assisted Living Guide and Checklist.")

American Association of Retired Persons
601 E Street NW
Washington,DC 20049
888-687-2277
Go to www.aarp.org and click on "Checklist for choosing assisted living."

Consumer Consortium on Assisted Living
2342 Oak Street
Falls Church, VA 22046
703-533-8121

http://www.ccal.org/bookstore.htm
(For purchase of a $14.95 video, "Choosing Assisted Living
. . . What You Need to Know.")

Dignity First® Training Questions for Facilities

Try to get specifics, not just general answers. Ask for a
list of topics that have been used to train staff. Are there
outcome measures for training? The probability is low
that you will get answers to many of these questions,
but just asking them will let the facility know you are an
informed consumer.

1. What dementia care training is required?

2. What are the topics in the training?

3. How is the dementia care training provided?
   (classroom lecture, afternoon inservice, reading
   materials, video, online)

4. Who provides the training?

5. Is there additional training for staff in the dementia/
   memory care unit?

6. How would I request training for staff if there is a
   special problem with my loved one?

7. Are all new staff members trained, and in what
   period of time after they start working?

PUBLICATIONS

Mace, Nancy L. and Rabins, Peter V. *The 36-Hour Day:
A Family Guide to Caring for Persons with Alzheimer
Disease, Related Dementing Illnesses, and Memory
Loss in Later Life*, 4th Ed. Baltimore: Johns Hopkins
University Press, 2006.

Coste, Joanne K. *Learning to Speak Alzheimer's: A Groundbreaking Approach for Everyone Dealing with the Disease.* Boston: Houghton Mifflin Harcourt, 2004.

Strauss, Claudia J. *Talking to Alzheimer's: Simple Ways to Connect with a Family Member or Friend.* Oakland, CA: New Harbinger, 2002.

Smith, Patricia B., Kenan, Mary M., and Kunic, Mark Edwin. *Alzheimer's for Dummies.* Hoboken, NJ: John Wiley & Sons, 2003.

CAREGIVER ASSISTANCE AND ORGANIZATIONS

Today's Caregiver (magazine)
3350 Griffin Road
Ft. Lauderdale, FL. 33312
800-829-0550
http://www.caregiver.com
(Resources for Alzheimer's caregivers and information about long-term care)

Family Caregiver Alliance
180 Montgomery Street
Suite 1100
San Francisco, CA 94104
800-445-8106
http://www.caregiver.org
(Includes a state-by-state guide of resources)

Department of Health and Human Services, Administration on Aging:
Administration on Aging
Washington, DC 20201

202 619-0724
http://www.aoa.gov (Click on "Elders & Families")

Alzheimer's Association
24/7 Helpline
tel: 1.800.272.3900
tdd: 1.866.403.3073
http://www.alz.org (Links to local associations)

Alzheimer's Foundation of America
322 8th Ave., 7th Fl.
New York, NY 10001
866-232-8484
http://www.alzfdn.org
(Provides education and support)

National Family Caregivers Association
10400 Connecticut Avenue, Suite 500
Kensington, MD 20895-3944
Toll Free: 1-800-896-3650
http://www.thefamilycaregiver.org
(Includes resources for caregivers of those with disabilities
and chronic illnesses, has links to two other sites: National
Alliance for Caregiving and Family Caregiving 101)

Consumer Consortium on Assisted Living
2342 Oak Street
Falls Church, VA 22046
703-533-8121
http://www.ccal.org/bookstore.htm
(Non-profit organization that focuses on consumer issues
in assisted living)

Assisted Living Consumer Alliance

Contact Eric Carlson of the National Senior Citizens Law Center, (213) 674-2813

http://www.assistedlivingconsumers.org (National organization that grew out of the National Citizen's Coalition for Nursing Home Reform [NCCNHR] and focuses on consumers and advocates)

American Association of Retired Persons

601 E Street NW
Washington,DC 20049
888-687-2277
http://assets.aarp.org/www.aarp.org (Click on "Assisted Living")

The Association for Frontotemporal Dementias

1616 Walnut Street, Suite 1100
Philadelphia, PA 19103
866-507-7222
http://www.ftd-picks.org

Lewy Body Dementia Association, Inc.

912 Killian Hill Road SW, Suite 202C
Lilburn, GA 30047
Caregiver Helpline: 800.539.9767
http://www.lbda.org

National Stroke Association:

National Stroke Association
9707 E Easter Lane Building B
Centennial, CO 80112
1(800)787.6537
http://www.stroke.org

National Parkinson Foundation:
1501 N.W. 9th Avenue / Bob Hope Road
Miami, Florida 33136-1494
Toll Free National: 1-800-327-4545
http://www.parkinson.org

National Association of Professional Geriatric Care Managers
3275 West Ina Road, Suite 130
Tucson, AZ 85741-2198
(520) 881-8008
http://www.caremanager.org
(Provides links to find a manager in your area)

National Hospice and Palliative Care Organization
1731 King Street, Suite 100
Alexandria, Virginia 22314
703/837-1500 (phone)
http://www.nhpco.org
(Provides information and education about end-of-life care)

INFORMATION AND ADVOCACY

The National Citizens' Coalition for Nursing Home Reform
1828 L Street, NS
Suite 801
Washington, DC 20036
202-332-2275
http://www.nccnhr.org (Coalition comprised of consumers and advocates; has information about assisted living)

Center for Excellence in Assisted Living
2342 Oak Street

Falls Church, VA 22046
202-465-1893
http://www.theceal.org
(Non-profit collaboration of national organizations; includes state-by-state information about regulations)

Pioneer Network
P.O. Box 18648
Rochester, New York 14618
(585) 271-7570 phone
http://www.pioneernetwork.net
(Advocacy network for providers and consumers)

National Academy of Elder Law Attorneys
1577 Spring Hill Road, Suite 220
Vienna, VA 22182
(703) 942-5711
http://www.naela.org
(Provides resources for lawyers and legal associations)

National Senior Citizens Law Center
1444 Eye St., NW Suite 1100
Washington, DC 20005
(202) 289-6976
http://www.nsclc.org
(Focuses on legal rights of low-income elders and those with disabilities)

Administration on Aging's National Center on Elder Abuse
Center for Community Research and Services
University of Delaware
297 Graham Hall
Newark, DE 19716
302-831-3525

http://www.ncea.aoa.gov
(Provides links to state resources)

National Long-Term Care Ombudsman Resource Center
1828 L Street, NW suite 801
Washington, DC 20036
202-332-2275
http://www.ltcombudsman.org (Click on "Ombudsman Locator" for state links)

Hospice Patients Alliance
4680 Shank Street
Rockford, MI 49341
616-866-9127
http://www.hospicepatients.org
(Provides hospice regulations for each state as well as legal and advocacy information)

Hospice Association of America
228 Seventh Street, SE
Washington, DC 20003
202-546-4769
http://www.nahc.org/haa
(An industry organization, but has Consumer Information section)

ASSISTED LIVING INDUSTRY GROUPS

Assisted Living Federation of America
1650 King St Ste 602
Alexandria, VA 22314-2747
703-894-1805
http://www.alfa.org

(National association for professionals operating assisted living facilities for elders)

American Association of Homes and Services for the Aging

2519 Connecticut Avenue, NW
Washington, D.C. 20008-1520
(202) 783-2242
http://www.aahsa.org
(National association for non-profit providers of senior care)

National Center for Assisted Living

1201 L Street, N.W.
Washington,D.C. 20005
202.842.4444
http://www.ncal.org
(Assisted living organization for the American Health Care Association [AHCA])

American Assisted Living Nurses Association

P.O. Box 10469
Napa, CA 94581
(707) 253-7299
http://www.alnursing.org
(Non-profit organization for nurses in assisted living)

COUNSELING/MENTAL HEALTH

The American Psychological Association

750 First Street, NE
Washington, DC 20002-4242
(800) 374-2721
http://apa.org
(Click on "Find a Psychologist")

American Association for Geriatric Psychiatry
7910 Woodmont Ave
Suite 1050
Bethesda, MD 20814-3004
301-654-7850
http://www.aagpgpa.org (Click on Patients and Caregivers)

The American Psychiatric Association
1000 Wilson Boulevard
Suite 1825
Arlington, VA 22209
1-888-35-77924
http://www.psych.org

The American Counseling Association
5999 Stevenson Ave.
Alexandria, VA 22304
(800) 347-6647
http://www.counseling.org

Mental health provider organizations
Mir Internet Marketing, Inc.
ATTN: FindCounseling.com
818 Harrison Street, Suite 205
Oak Park, Illinois 60304
Phone: (708) 434-2260
http://www.findcounseling.com
(Click on "Mental Health Resources" to find all types of mental health provider organizations by state)

APPENDIX B.

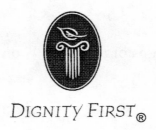

DIGNITY FIRST®

BRAINWORK: UNDERSTANDING ALZHEIMER'S FROM THE GROUND UP

Martha E. Leatherman, MD
Katherine E. Goethe, PhD

INTRODUCTION: WHAT IS IN THE BRAIN AND HOW IT WORKS

The Neuron: Or Your Brain Is Not Just a Mass of Goo

Some people are aware that Alzheimer's disease is a brain disorder of some kind, but the most commonly asked question is probably, "What exactly is Alzheimer's disease?" This appendix answers this question as well as the second and third most frequently asked questions, "What causes the disease?" and "How is it diagnosed?"

To understand the answers, some basic knowledge of the brain and how it functions is required. The information about the brain and brain function is technical, but **stick with it**, because after you understand this, you will grasp more than many health professionals about this complex set of diseases.

At the outset of this chapter, we must humbly beg our scientific colleagues' pardon for oversimplification. We are also aware that many details and hypotheses have been omitted, since the purpose of this appendix is simply to present a conceptual overview of brain function.

Most people know that the brain is enclosed in the skull and that it is somehow associated with blood and some sort of "goo." People may have heard of "gray matter" and "white matter," but don't really understand what exactly is in the brain. Well, the brain is really composed of millions of nerve cells called *neurons* (the gray matter and white matter) bathed in a clear fluid called *cerebrospinal fluid* or *CSF*. There are blood vessels running all around and through the brain to bring the neurons necessary nutrients and oxygen to keep them alive. Below is a picture of a generic neuron:

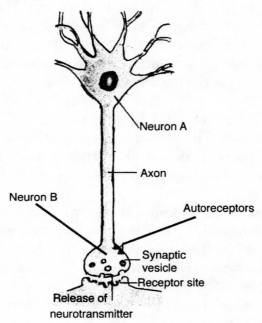

The term "generic" is used because, like people, neurons come in many shapes and sizes. However, for purposes of illustration, the neuron above is representative enough for us to understand some basic facts. One way to think of the neuron is as a computer with a cable going in and a cable going out. The *dendrite* is the cable in and the *axon* is the cable out. The cell body is the computer itself. The information carried through these cables is carried in the form of little packets of chemicals called *neurotransmitters.*

There are many neurotransmitters, but three important ones for our discussion are *norepinephrine* (NE), *dopamine* (DA), and *acetylcholine* (Ach). Each neuron makes a specific kind of neurotransmitter. The neurotransmitter is manufactured in the cell body, and then it travels down the axon where it is released into the *synaptic cleft,* which is the space between the axon of the first neuron and the dendrite of the next one. The neurotransmitter packet is then "picked up" by the *receptor* on the dendrite of the receiving neuron, where it starts a chain of chemical reactions in the cell body and makes the receiving neuron "do" something— typically either "turn on" (*excite*) or "turn off" (*inhibit*) the next neuron. The process acts sort of like a relay race where the baton (i.e. the neurotransmitter) is passed, along with instructions about what the receiving neuron should do next.

It's important to know that a neuron cannot obey just any neurotransmitter. The neuron has to have the right kind of receptors in order to make sense of what the transmitter is trying to tell it. Some neurons have receptors for NE, some for DA, and some for Ach. It's almost like a lock (receptor) and key (neurotransmitter). Or, thinking in terms of our computer analogy, it is not enough just to plug a cable into a computer and expect to have it work. The electrical cable bringing in electricity from the power source must be plugged into the proper inlet to the computer. Likewise, the phone cord must be plugged into the properly corresponding receptacle on the computer. If you tried to connect to the Internet by plugging your power cord into the phone port on your computer, you would not have any success. So, we see that the three components of neuron function are inextricably coordinated and work together to send the signals necessary for brain function: a neuritic dendrite, the neurotransmitter itself, and the receptor.

The drawing below is a schematic drawing of the three components. The space between the axon of the sending neuron and the dendrite of the receiving neuron is called the *synaptic cleft* and is the area across which the neurotransmitter packet travels to reach the axon of the next neurotransmitter.

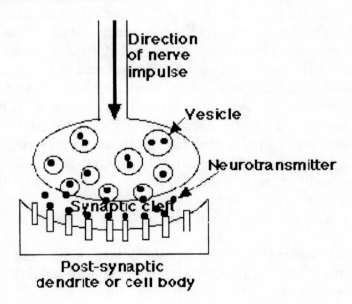

Direction
of nerve
impulse

Vesicle

Neurotransmitter

Synaptic cleft

Post-synaptic
dendrite or cell body

OK, so now you understand the basic synapse. Let's follow a neurotransmitter through its path. Use the illustration on page 147 to help you follow along. We will use acetylcholine (Ach) because that is the neurotransmitter most commonly discussed in Alzheimer's dementia. Neuronal cell A produces Ach and stores it in packets *(vesicles)* in its axon. Neurons send messages to each other, so when neuron A receives instructions to do so, it releases these vesicles into the synaptic cleft where they migrate to the receptors designed for them on the dendrites of neuron B. Much like putting the correct key in a particular lock, the Ach molecules bind to the receptors on neuron B, thus initiating a chain of biochemical events that causes neuron B to "do" its job—whatever that might be.

Now, how does neuron A know when it's released enough Ach? In the drawing of the neuron above, look at those receptors on the axon of the neuron A—they are called *autoreceptors* and they also bind to Ach. When the Ach binds to the autoreceptors, they *inhibit,* or turn off the production of Ach. As the concentration of Ach in the synaptic cleft diminishes, the number of autoreceptors that are filled with Ach also diminishes and so the neuron resumes production of the neurotransmitter. Another way the body regulates the amount of neurotransmitter floating around is by using an enzyme present in the synaptic cleft called *acetylcholinesterase* which *degrades* or chews up Ach. This can be compared to a "cleanup crew" to dispense of waste. So now we have a mechanism for production, a mechanism to stop production, and a mechanism to degrade the neurotransmitter in the synaptic cleft.

You should know that the above explanation is extremely simplified and is merely a way to give you a conceptual understanding of the communication between single neurons. In reality, there are multiple neurotransmitter systems, as well as second messengers, enzymes, and large networks of neurons. Sometimes the same neurotransmitter can inhibit one neuron and excite another depending on what kind of receptor is activated.

You might have heard of a "chemical imbalance" in the brain. Well, all these biochemicals from the receptors to the neurotransmitters to the enzymes must work together in an amazing degree of complexity, and any "break" in the system (neuroscientists call this a *perturbation*) will cause the system to work improperly. Also, remember since these neurons are part of complex networks, a perturbation in one area will likely affect neuronal networks in distant areas of the brain. For instance, if gasoline tankers cannot get into a city for a prolonged time, the transport of plastic milk bottles made at the factories in the city will slow down. The result would be that in other towns, the dairies would be unable to bottle milk, and would have to slow production, decreasing the availability of milk to consumers. From this analogy, you can see how the chain of events could go on and on. This kind of chaining is precisely what happens in the brain.

ALZHEIMER'S AND DEMENTIA

WHAT DOES THE BRAIN HAVE TO DO WITH ALZHEIMER'S?

Well, now that you have an understanding of basic neuroscience, what does this have to do with Alzheimer's? Remember that we said earlier that Ach is the neurotransmitter commonly implicated in Alzheimer's. Well, nothing is as simple as it seems on the surface, but for purposes of understanding this conceptual framework, it is true that we currently believe Ach is an integral neurotransmitter involved in Alzheimer's dementia. On its most basic level, Alzheimer's is caused by the death of the neurons that make Ach. When these neurons die, they can't make Ach and without Ach, the neurons that depend on Ach to carry out their own jobs, aren't able to function. This in itself is problematic enough, but the absence of Ach can allow other neurotransmitters, such as NE and DA, to act unopposed, without the degree of inhibition necessary for regulation of complex functions such as thinking and remembering.

Alzheimer's Dementia

Alzheimer's disease is one disease among many known as the *dementias*. Strictly speaking, dementia is a very general term that describes changes in brain function marked by changes in behavior and thinking (*cognition*). There are many different causes for the changes in the brain which cause dementia, and with a very few exceptions, they are irreversible.

While there are over 50 different kinds of dementia, common to all these different forms of dementia, including Alzheimer's, is the fact that neurons are damaged. These damaged neurons disrupt the normal way the brain functions and when the brain can't do its job, the afflicted person will experience thinking, behavioral, emotional or movement problems—and often a combination of all of these.

The most common form of dementia is Alzheimer's disease, which was first described and characterized in 1906 by Dr. Alois Alzheimer and his colleague Dr. Emile Kraeplin. The disease was named "Alzheimer's dementia" (rather than "Kreaplin's dementia") because Dr. Kraeplin believed that the visible brain changes that Dr. Alzheimer saw under the microscope were of such importance that the disease should carry the name "Alzheimer." Of course at that time, neither Dr. Alzheimer nor Dr. Kraeplin knew the cause of the disease, but Dr. Alzheimer's classic descriptions of the brain changes and behavior of afflicted patients crystallized our recognition of the disease, and ultimately improved our understanding of other dementias.

Diagnosis: How Do You Know It's Alzheimer's?

In the past, it was the rule that Alzheimer's was only formally diagnosed by brain biopsy or autopsy. Now, thanks to new technology, a better understanding of the disease, and especially because we have medications that can help slow its progression, we usually make the diagnosis of Alzheimer's disease *clinically* which just means that we look at a person's symptoms, make sure the symptoms are not due to other identifiable causes, and then, based on the symptom pattern we see, make a diagnosis. This process of clinical diagnosis sounds simple and straightforward. However, although it may be simple, it's far from easy. As you will see in the discussion below, the symptoms of Alzheimer's disease are similar to those of many other forms of dementia, but can usually be distinguished by a skilled clinician using careful physical, neurological, and neuropsychological examination techniques.

Alzheimer's specialists can accurately diagnose Alzheimer's disease about 90% of the time. The diagnostic process includes a complete medical history, examination, and laboratory testing. The medical history should include questions about family history, psychiatric problems or symptoms, physical complaints, all the medications a person is taking, habits such as alcohol or drug use, and memory symptoms. Usually, in order to make sure the medical history is as accurate as possible, a physician will enlist the aid of a family member or spouse.

A number of other illnesses can mimic the symptoms of Alzheimer's, and so it's important to use a physical examination, laboratory, and imaging studies to *rule out* or exclude other treatable causes of the symptoms of dementia. Some of these conditions include depression, dehydration, *hypothyroidism* (or "low thyroid"), B12 deficiency, syphilis, urinary tract infection, or low sodium in the blood. In order to look for these other medical problems, physicians utilize medical tests including urinalysis, complete blood count (CBC), full blood chemistry profile (such as sodium, potassium, glucose), thyroid function tests (T3,T4, and TSH), test for syphilis, vitamin B12 and folate levels. Because brain tumors and strokes can cause symptoms similar to Alzheimer's, some form of brain imaging such as CT or MRI is often necessary when making the diagnosis of dementia.

Neuropsychological testing might be recommended in which a specialized psychologist with expert understanding of brain function as well as human behavior will administer an extensive series of mental tests designed to identify and characterize changes in memory, judgment, insight, and planning. Some physicians, particularly geriatric psychiatrists and certain neurologists, might not routinely need full neuropsychological testing. However, regardless of who is doing the examination, any patient with suspected Alzheimer's should undergo a careful clinical examination of thinking or *mental status examination*. Sometimes, in the hands of a skilled physician, patients and families might not even notice that the majority of the mental status examination is taking place because the physician is able to weave the examination questions into conversation. Sometimes physicians are criticized by patients and families who don't understand this. The physician is perceived as "just talking and joking" with the patient. In reality, that "talking and joking" is the mark of a sophisticated clinician.

Although it is tempting to look at a list of symptoms associated with Alzheimer's and try to "diagnose" yourself, and although lists of warning signs to be aware of exist, the diagnosis of Alzheimer's is simply not possible to make using a check-off list. As we said earlier, diagnosing mental, cognitive, or behavioral problems is simple (there are no invasive tests, few laboratory tests, and a relatively small number of symptoms), but not easy. Not all memory loss is Alzheimer's just as not all fever is the flu. Another way to conceptualize this is to think of how we might identify the different year models of two red cars by the same manufacturer. Both have wheels, a steering wheel, seats, a hood, windows, and headlights. Both might even be the same size, have the same number of doors, and be convertibles. An auto enthusiast would know, possibly at a glance or after some examination, which was the 1957 and which was the 1961 model. Knowing nothing about cars, you might never identify the model year simply by checking off the various features of the cars. The ability to identify the model year depends not only on recognizing the cars' features, but also the subtle differences in those features as well as the ways they are arranged on the cars. Similarly, patients with Alzheimer's and Lewy Body dementia both have memory loss, thinking problems, may have hallucinations and mood changes, but the two diseases are distinctly different.

Given the above caution about diagnosis of dementia, we will briefly discuss some of the cardinal features of Alzheimer's dementia. For most people, the hallmark of Alzheimer's disease is loss of memory. While this is mostly true, Alzheimer's specialists know that not all memory loss is Alzheimer's or even dementia. In fact, people are often surprised to realize how much of the distant past a patient with early Alzheimer's can remember. Family members will often comment, "Her memory for the past is great, so I don't think she has Alzheimer's." In fact, the memory disturbance that is the hallmark of Alzheimer's is *short-term* memory loss. We like to emphasize to people that this short-term memory loss is best understood as the inability to learn new material. For example, a patient with Alzheimer's might absolutely believe that his wallet was stolen because he can't remember (or learn) that he gave it to his son for safekeeping. No amount of arguing will help, because for the patient with Alzheimer's disease, the new information doesn't "stick." This is very important to understand when considering the best ways to interact with people with Alzheimer's. Besides memory loss, the symptoms a physician looks for when making a diagnosis of Alzheimer's disease include poor sequencing and planning, poor judgment, *apathy* or loss of initiative, poor insight, trouble with location and directions and confusion.

Another common misconception about Alzheimer's is that of "alertness." We will often hear health care workers confidently assert that a patient doesn't have Alzheimer's because he is "alert and not confused." Level of alertness describes to what extent someone is awake or aroused—not the degree of confusion or memory loss. In fact, "confusion" is often not apparent in a person with dementia. A person with dementia might appear to be very clear minded and not perplexed or disordered at all. However, with careful observation, it will become evident that the person is not in possession of important facts such as day, year, or situation. A problem occurs when we try to identify dementia solely by observing a person's behavior. Many people are able to successfully hide their memory and thinking problems for long periods of time because their social skills such as conversational ability are still intact. One way to think about this is to remember a time you have been at a party and someone comes up to you and says, "Hi! Do you remember me?" If you don't remember, you can still carry on a reasonable conversation for ten or so minutes by "covering" the fact that you don't remember. No one watching would say you were "confused," but the fact remains that you are clueless as to whom you are talking! This is an example of using social skills to cover memory lapse, and many people with Alzheimer's and other dementias continue to have good social skills long into the progression of their illnesses. So we see that merely relying on external cues such as "alertness" or "confusion" to detect dementia can be very misleading.

Other than brain biopsy, (which, of course, is not recommended),there is no single test that pinpoints a diagnosis of Alzheimer's disease. Brain tissue of someone with Alzheimer's disease when examined under a microscope shows characteristic "plaques and tangles," but these microscopic findings are found in the brains of some older people who don't have Alzheimer's disease. Later in the disease, imaging studies such as MRI and CT show brain shrinkage, but none of these test results is unique to Alzheimer's. They must be correlated with mental, physical and laboratory examination in order to make the diagnosis.

No discussion of Alzheimer's disease diagnosis would be complete without looking at the genetic defects associated with the disease. There seem to be two main categories of Alzheimer's disease: early-onset and late-onset. Early-onset Alzheimer's disease tends to run in families and to be associated with abnormalities or mutations in several genes. The most common is *presenilin 1 (PS1)*. There is genetic testing available for this gene, but it is not much used in clinical practice, and there are ethical and legal implications for that testing. Public policy considerations involved with genetic testing are beyond the scope of this book, but, to give you one example, suppose that you found you had the "Alzheimer's" gene and later developed Alzheimer's disease. Your health insurance company could then decide that you had a "pre-existing condition" and refuse coverage for medical care.

The genetic abnormality most clearly associated with late-onset Alzheimer's disease is the *apolipoprotein epsilon 4 (ApoE4)* gene. We must remember that at this point, the ApoE4 gene is only a risk factor. That means that in people with the gene, the risk for Alzheimer's disease is higher, but that not everyone with the gene will get the disease. We do not yet know the triggers required to switch the ApoE4 gene over (turn it on, in other words) to begin the Alzheimer's disease process. We also do not know why some people with the gene get the disease and others do not.

WHAT CAUSES DEMENTIA?

As you will recall from the discussion above, many different diseases can cause dementia, but what actually happens to cause those neurons to die? Well, we don't know all the reasons neurons die, but there are a few common underlying conditions that can damage the brain.

Vascular Changes

Remember that neurons in the brain are surrounded by a huge network of blood vessels. The blood vessels called *arteries* carry oxygen and nutrients to the brain and blood vessels called *veins* carry waste products away from the brain. Some of these blood vessels are large enough to be seen without a microscope while others, called *capillaries* are so narrow that only one red blood cell can pass through at a time. Now, a huge amount of work is done by the capillaries in the brain. Because the capillaries are so tiny, oxygen carried by the red blood cells can easily leave the capillary by seeping or *diffusing* across the very thin capillary wall. From there, the oxygen can enter the nerve cell to supply its needs. In the same way, waste in the form of carbon dioxide can leave the neuron and enter the capillary where the red blood cell takes it away so the body can dispose of it. Likewise, other nutrients carried in the blood can enter the neuron and other neuronal wastes can be removed.

In people with *atherosclerosis* or "hardening of the arteries," the inside of the arteries is coated in places with beads of fatty deposits. This coating causes the arteries to become narrower—like a clogged drain. As these fatty deposits build up, the body tries to cover them with scar tissue. Unfortunately, this scar tissue further narrows the arteries and it also *calcifies* or develops a crusty, jagged coating inside the blood vessel. When blood flows through this rough artery, clotting cells in the blood called *platelets* bump against the jagged edges and release chemicals that cause the blood to clot in the artery at the area of the calcification. At this point, no more blood can get through the narrow artery or capillary—sort of like a clogged drain that has a tissue stuck in it. The neurons downstream of this clogged capillary or artery do not get the oxygen or nutrients they need and so they start to die. Similar to a hair that is singed, these neurons "frizzle up" and completely lose the character of a neuron. They can no longer function. If this happens at places all over the brain, enough brain tissue can be affected that you have generalized problems with thinking and behavior. When they die, neurons release all sorts of chemicals, some of which are actually almost corrosive and in turn damage surrounding, healthy neurons. We call this corrosive action *inflammation*. In addition, the body's defense system starts working, and white blood cells rush to the area to try to clean up the mess. The end result is that surrounding neurons become affected by the toxins, inflammatory products, and white blood cells in the area and so finally you have a small area—usually microscopic—consisting of many damaged neurons.

Strokes, Mini-Strokes, and TIA's

Most of us have heard of strokes. Many of us have heard of "mini-strokes," and a few of us have heard of "TIA's." Just what are these and what do they have to do with dementia? Well, in order to really understand these three processes, we have to start with a mental picture. Think of a city water supply. All of the lawns (neurons) in the city depend on the flow of water to survive in a drought. If the main water supply to the city is cut off long enough, all the lawns will die. If the supply to an entire neighborhood is cut off, the lawns in that neighborhood die. If the water to a single house is cut off, only one lawn will die.

Now, if we consider the water lines to be the blood vessels, we can see how this might work in the brain. If one of the major arteries supplying the brain is blocked long enough, a large area of the brain will die. *Ischemia* is a word that describes the interruption of the blood supply and oxygen to body tissue. We have all heard of people who have had a "major stroke" which leaves them unable to move an entire half of their body. This is usually due to brain ischemia from the blockage of a major artery which supplies blood to a large area of the brain. Millions of nerve cells die, and there is a huge inflammatory process in the surrounding neurons. Often, inflammation gets better over time, and that's one reason that people with strokes regain some function over the few weeks following a stroke.

Of course, not all strokes leave people paralyzed over half of their bodies. We can see, using our water supply analogy, why this is so. If the water supply to a neighborhood gets cut off, the lawns in that neighborhood will die. This is like a stroke in only one fairly small area of the brain. If the water supply gets cut off to only one house, only the grass at that house dies. In the brain we would call this a "mini-stroke," which is the blockage of a tiny venule or network of capillaries (*capillary bed*). You would need sophisticated imaging like a powerful MRI to see the damage in a mini-stroke. Imagine, however, that water supply to single houses is blocked in multiple areas across the city maybe one or two houses on each block. Taken one by one, there might not be much of an effect on the city as a whole. Taken together, though, the total damage to the city is great. This is the real danger in mini-strokes. If one capillary or venule is vulnerable to blockage because of atherosclerosis, then all of the small vessels are also vulnerable, and chances are that there are many blockages at multiple areas in the brain. When all of these small areas die, and usually it happens a little bit at a time, there is a major change in function of the brain. Usually we won't see a sudden dramatic result like the weakness of an arm or leg, but we will see a slow change in thinking ability, or a gradual decline in the ability to verbalize things, or gradual onset of balance problems. Over time, as the damage accumulates, the person can become quite debilitated. In fact, a person with lots of mini-strokes usually displays symptoms almost identical to Alzheimer's.

A TIA or *transient ischemic attack* is similar to a mini-stroke except that, by definition, a TIA is not permanent. The blood supply to an area of the brain is only temporarily (transiently) interrupted. The body's ability to dissolve blood clots works well enough that the blockage breaks free before the neurons die completely. Using our lawn analogy to try to understand a TIA, we can see that when the water is cut off to a house or a neighborhood, the grass begins to wilt. When the water is turned back on, the grass perks up again. Since the grass was never without water long enough to die, when it gets water, it can be revived. The thing about TIA's is that the underlying process that causes the blockage is continual and so you can have more TIA's and the next one might not be reversed by the body in time, so you would have a mini-stroke or stroke. Also, because the underlying process—atherosclerosis—is ongoing, you are at higher risk for a major stroke.

By this point, you are most likely asking how anyone can know the difference between "mini-strokes" and Alzheimer's if the two look so similar clinically. Well, in fact dedicated scientists working on unraveling the mysteries of Alzheimer's are looking at whether ischemia might actually set off a sequence of events in the brain (perhaps involving inflammation) that provokes or perhaps accelerates Alzheimer's. As you have seen above, loss of blood supply is one cause of neuronal death, and is responsible for vascular (or multi-infarct) dementia. What, though, causes the preferential damage to acetylcholine (*cholinergic*) neurons in the brains of people with Alzheimer's? Unfortunately, we don't know for sure. There are a number of findings in the brains of Alzheimer's patients that have given researchers clues as to the cause of neuronal death, and we will discuss a few of them below.

Factors Associated with neuronal Death in Alzheimer's Disease

The Amyloid Hypothesis

According to the Alzheimer's Association, the amyloid hypothesis is the most popular hypothesis among researchers today, and the most common request for grants from the Alzheimer's Association is to study the amyloid hypothesis. As we discussed above there are characteristic "plaques" and "tangles" seen under a microscope in the brain tissue of Alzheimer's patients. The plaques are more specifically called "amyloid plaques." The theory linking these plaques to Alzheimer's goes something like this: there is a common protein found in the brain called amyloid precursor protein (APP). We don't know the function of this protein, but part of it is cut by an enzyme to make the substance called amyloid. If it is cut improperly by the body, it causes an unstable piece to be formed called beta-amyloid which is sort of sticky and clumps together to form amyloid plaques which interfere with neuronal functioning. These plaques "gum up the works" so to speak. While there is a lot of evidence linking amyloid plaques and Alzheimer's, some scientists believe that the amyloid plaque is simply a protective mechanism the body employs to attempt to minimize damage from the real culprit in Alzheimer's disease. [1] The analogy would be that the bump on your finger is not the cause of the pain you feel, the bump is formed in response to the splinter embedded in the tissue below the bump. These scientists point to the puzzling finding that many elderly adults without Alzheimer's or other dementias have amyloid plaques and that maybe in these individuals, the plaques were there not because they caused the disease, but because they did their proper job of protecting the neurons from whatever biological process was threatening them.

The Tau Theory

This is the theory which enjoys the place of second prominence in Alzheimer's research today. The Tau theory addresses the formation of the neurofibrillary tangles ("frizzles" described above) found in the brains of patients with Alzheimer's. The research being done in this area explores the possible mechanism by which *tau* (another protein essential to the proper functioning of cells) is deformed and damaged. These damaged tau proteins eventually lead to the formation of neurofibrillary tangles. Again, the question becomes "Why are these tau proteins deformed? What damages them?" There might be some association between the formation of these damaged proteins and the presence of the ApoE 4 gene, and some have proposed a theory called the *amyloid cascade* in which neurofibrillary tangles are formed as part of a deterioration process that starts with amyloid plaques.[2] Again, though, what causes the initial abnormality that starts this process? Why do some people have these brain abnormalities and others don't? We don't know the answers to these questions. Unfortunately, still haven't found out what actually causes Alzheimer's.

Inflammation Theory

Scientists have noted that in patients regularly taking anti-inflammatory medications such as ibuprofen, the rate of Alzheimer's is much lower than expected. This observation has led to research focusing on whether or not anti-oxidants (which relieve inflammation) and other anti-inflammatory medications will reduce the symptoms of Alzheimer's disease. Another avenue of research dealing with inflammation is that of the connection between Alzheimer's disease and other known inflammatory conditions. Perhaps changes associated with atherosclerosis (described above) lead to inflammation which then "turns on" the amyloid cascade discussed above. These are all exciting theories, but will take years to investigate.

Free Radicals

When chemical processes take place in a cell, waste products are produced. Some of these waste products are toxic to cells. One group of these toxic compounds is called the *free radicals*. Our bodies naturally employ mechanisms to get rid of or *clear* free radicals. However, there is some thought that as the body ages, its intrinsic mechanism for neutralizing these free radicals becomes inefficient, so the free radicals damage nearby healthy cells. In addition, as we discussed above, when there is loss of oxygen to the neurons and resultant damage, free radicals are formed.

L-Glutamate

L-glutamate is an amino acid found in the human body. In the central nervous system, it is what is called an *excitatory* amino acid. This means that it can act like a neurotransmitter and "turn on" or excite nerve cells. It does this using a receptor called the N-methyl-D-aspartate (NMDA) receptor. There are NMDA receptors on almost all the neurons in the central nervous system. The l-glutamate hypothesis suggests that too much excitation of the NMDA receptor causes damage to the neuron and might cause the neuronal damage associated with Alzheimer's disease.

The Insulin Hypothesis

We have known for a long time about the increased risk of stroke and vascular dementia in people with diabetes. Diabetes causes narrowing of the small arteries and arterioles all over the body, and that includes the brain. As you will recall from our discussion of vascular dementia above, narrow arteries can cause the body to have difficulty in supplying oxygen and nutrients to the brain and so the brain is at risk of damage. What is very interesting, though, is the connection between diabetes and Alzheimer's.

For years, scientists have been puzzled by the role diabetes plays in Alzheimer's. Although we know that the risk of vascular dementia and stroke is greater for people with diabetes, the role of diabetes and insulin in Alzheimer's has been unclear. Some studies have shown a connection between Alzheimer's and diabetes, some studies have shown that Alzheimer's is found **less** often in people with diabetes (in fact, some scientists have opined that diabetes and Alzheimer's are "mutually exclusive"), [3,4,5,6] and some studies have been inconclusive.

Now as we discussed earlier, there is a possible role for diabetes in both the beginning and the progression of Alzheimer's due to its effects on the blood vessels of the brain. However, there might actually be an independent role for insulin itself in causing the neuronal damage associated with Alzheimer's that is completely separate from its effects on blood vessels. We are beginning to unravel this mystery by looking at the many complex actions that brain glucose and insulin have on memory.

Insulin affects processes all over the body by attaching to specific insulin receptors (remember the "locks and keys?") located on cells throughout the body. There are also insulin receptors found in brain cells that enable the brain to utilize glucose efficiently. There are even insulin receptors in the synapses in the brain that are known to participate in the regulation of two important neurotransmitters, gamma-aminobuytric acid (GABA) and N-methyl-D-aspartate (NMDA). [7]

Now, sometimes cells are *insulin resistant,* which means that the normal attachment of the insulin to the cell causes only a weak response from the cell instead of the normal response. We see this in people who have *Type II* or *non-insulin dependent diabetes.* This means that these people produce plenty of insulin (in contrast to *Type I* or *insulin dependent diabetes*), but because of the poorly functioning receptors, the cells can't use the insulin present in the body. In that case, the body produces more and more insulin to try to ramp up the cellular response.

So, what does this have to do with Alzheimer's? Well, interestingly enough there are a number of investigators who have noticed connections among the way glucose is metabolized in the brain, insulin's actions in the brain, memory and Alzheimer's disease. It also seems that the effects of glucose on memory are in some way dependent on how sensitive, or efficient, the insulin receptors are in directing how glucose is metabolized. In fact, animal studies have shown that the presence of high levels of insulin in the brain for long periods of time as well as fluctuations in blood glucose worsen memory. [8]

Clinical studies in humans have also shown that patients with Alzheimer's disease are more likely than healthy older adults to have reduced insulin sensitivity, and further suggest that apolipoprotein E genotype (we discussed that in the genetics section above) may influence the effects of insulin on glucose, memory, and amyloid precursor protein processing. Taken together, these findings support an association among Alzheimer's disease, impaired glucose metabolism, and reduced insulin sensitivity.

In humans, then, it appears that the combination of age, presence of ApoE and insulin resistance might increase the risk of Alzheimer's, but we are still a long way from knowing whether these are the only factors or even what level of risk each factor might contribute.

Scientists are working to find the cause for the plaques and tangles associated with Alzheimer's. There is no definite answer to the question of what causes these brain abnormalities or Alzheimer's disease. It could be that what we now call "Alzheimer's" is in reality a group of similar diseases with disparate mechanisms. It could be that a combination of some or all of the mechanisms discussed above could influence the development of Alzheimer's. It could be that there are processes responsible for Alzheimer's which we have not yet even dreamed of—much less discovered.

REFERENCES

1. Lee HG, Casadesus G, Zhu X, Takeda A, Perry G, Smith MA: Challenging the amyloid cascade hypothesis: senile plaques and amyloid-beta as protective adaptations to Alzheimer's disease. *Annals of the New York Academy of Science.* 2004 Jun; 1019:1-4.

2. Huang HC, Jiang ZF: Accumulated amyloid-beta peptide and hyperphosphorylated tau protein: relationship and links in Alzheimer's disease. *Journal of Alzheimer's Disease.* 2009; 16(1):15-27

3. Wolf-Klein GP, Silverstone FA, Brod MS, et al.: Are Alzheimer patients healthier? *Journal of the American Geriatric Society.* 1988; 36:219-224.

4. Mortel KF, Wood S, Pavol MA, Meyer JS, Rexer JL: Analysis of familial and individual risk factors among patients with ischemic vascular dementia and Alzheimer's disease. *Angiology.* 1993; 44:599-605.

5. Landin K, Blennow K, Wallin A, Gottfries CG. Low blood pressure and blood glucose levels in Alzheimer's disease. Evidence for a hypometabolic disorder? *Journal of Internal Medicine.* 1993; 233:357-363.

6. Nielson KA, Nolan JH, Berchtold NC, Sanman CA, Mulnard RA, Cotman CO. Apolipoprotein-E genotyping of diabetic dementia patients: is diabetes rare in Alzheimer's disease? *Journal of the American Geriatric Society.* 1996; 44:897-904.

7. Gasparini L, Netzer WJ, Greengard P, Xu H. Does insulin dysfunction play a role in Alzheimer's disease? *Trends in Pharmacological Science.* 2002; 23:288-293.

8. Watson GS, Craft S. Modulation of memory by insulin and glucose: neuropsychological observations in Alzheimer's disease. *Current Drug Targets.* 2004; Aug; 5(6):565

APPENDIX C.

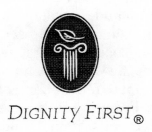

DIGNITY FIRST®

BRAINWORK: BRAIN FUNCTION AND BEHAVIOR

Martha E. Leatherman, MD
Katherine E. Goethe, PhD

As described in Appendix B, Alzheimer's disease and other dementias affect the entire brain, not just the areas that have to do with memory. Therefore, a basic understanding of how the brain functions is required to understand the behaviors of people with dementia.

First, let's consider that our brains get information from the world around us through five senses: seeing, hearing, tasting, smelling, and feeling/touching. Information gathered by the nerves in our sensory organs (our eyes, our ears, our taste buds, our nose, and our skin) is transmitted through the nervous system to the brain, which registers that data, processes it, and compares it with already stored information and knowledge. So if you think, "I would like to put on my shoes," your brain initiates that action by sending signals through the nervous system to the muscles in your arms, hands and feet, triggering the action of putting on shoes. But before any of that happens, you must see a shoe, recognize it as a shoe, and know what to do with it. Knowing what to do with that shoe requires that your brain possess sufficient organizational, problem-solving and decision-making functions of the brain and that all of those functions work together in unison to enable you to act. For instance, you need to be able to recognize and judge the correct shoes for the occasion, for the weather, and for your own feet.

It is very important to remember that the entire brain is interconnected, and communication between the various parts of the brain is crucial. Even though the brain is much more complex than the electrical wiring in your home, a brief look at the steps we take when a light doesn't turn on might help to explain the interdependency of various parts of the brain. You walk into a room, intending to turn on the lights, but when you flip the light switch, nothing happens. You assume that the light bulb in the lamp has burned out, so you change it. You flip the switch again, but nothing happens. You check the plug to make sure the lamp is plugged in. It is. You check the lights in other rooms and they are on, so you know the electrical power to the house isn't the problem. Likewise, you check the circuit breakers and discover that they are functioning properly, so you are left wondering if the wiring to that room is broken, or the wall plug is broken, or maybe the light switch itself is broken.

You can see from the above example that the symptom of the problem (the light bulb does not light up) is not necessarily the cause of the problem. You also notice that the cause of the lack of response of the light bulb might be something far-removed from the bulb itself. Similarly, if one part of the complex network of cells in your brain isn't communicating with another part, then distant areas of the brain can be affected, and might not even work, like the light bulb.

Neuropsychologists use such a logical, step-by-step method to figure out how the brain is functioning and what might be "broken." In a real-life example, let's say that you put a business letter down in front of someone who you know can see and hear, and you ask him to read it. He just sits there looking at you or at the letter. You might begin by wondering whether or not he can understand you. You do not know at this point whether he doesn't speak your language or his brain cannot process and understand oral language at all (*receptive aphasia*). Perhaps he does not recognize the letter you have just placed in front of him as being a letter (*visual recognition deficits*), or he cannot read (either illiteracy or acquired reading disability), or he cannot speak to you (*expressive aphasia*), or he can't initiate a movement to pick up the letter without a cue (*executive dysfunction*). In order to find out why he doesn't react to the letter, a neuropsychologist will test each of those skills until the cause of the problem is revealed.

Regrettably, most people are not aware of the multiple areas of neuronal damage in Alzheimer's disease. For that reason, caregivers are not equipped to understand the complex reasons why a person with Alzheimer's can't follow directions. What happens most often in Alzheimer's is that a person will not obey the instructions of the caregiver, and the caregiver will assume that the person is just not motivated or is being disobedient or stubborn. Because they do not understand the brain's complexities and functions, professional caregivers turn to us as "psychiatric experts" or "psychological experts" to provide counseling or medications to make the resident in assisted living more "obedient," regardless of the neurological or disease-driven cause of the behavior. This could often be avoided by a simple understanding of how the brain works or doesn't work in Alzheimer's.

This is akin to always blaming a burned out light bulb when a light won't turn on. Caregivers even get angry at persons with Alzheimer's if the caregiver "explains" and the person still doesn't follow the instructions. You might as well get angry at the light bulb.

Brain Regions

Now that you have an understanding of the general way that we look at brain function and how interconnected the brain is, let's look at the various regions of the brain in more detail. First of all, the brain is organized into two hemispheres, and each hemisphere has a subcortical portion, and a cortical portion as shown below. The cortex is shown as the cerebrum, and the *subcortex* is the lighter part in the middle of the figure, below the corpus collosum.

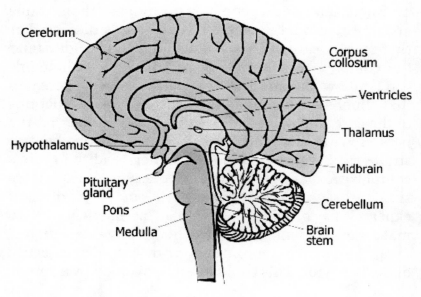

The brain is composed of millions of neurons, as you know from Appendix B. The gray portions are the outer portions of the brain, called the cortex. You have probably heard people described as "using their gray matter" when they think or have ideas.

The white matter of the brain is composed of the axons of the neurons (recall from Appendix B that the axon is the fiber along which the message is carried to the next neuron). The white matter and the brain structures in the middle and beneath the brain are referred to as *subcortex*. Here's where the communication part comes in. The cortex communicates with the subcortex, which sends messages back up to the cortex either back to the area from which the signal originated or to another distant area, and so on. Within the subcortex are deeper structures called the *thalamus*, the *hypothalamus*, and other areas that have to do with speech, memory, movement, and coordination. These deeper structures are almost like islands within the subcortex. The thalamus is similar to a Grand Central Station, where sensory information comes in and is transmitted to brain areas that can use it, and where information comes in from other areas of the brain for transmission. This is a very busy part of the brain, because it is constantly disseminating and transmitting information so your brain gets continuous, immediate messaging. The hypothalamus controls our basic functions of body temperature, thirst, hunger, and sexual arousal. It is also involved in behavior and mood. Because so many of the subcortical areas have to do with movement and control of our bodies (the *motor* functions), those people with subcortical dementias (for example dementia associated with Parkinson's disease) may have motor problems at the same time as their other cognitive difficulties. Even though Alzheimer's is classified as a type of "cortical dementia," in its more advanced stages of progressive neuronal destruction, it also affects subcortical areas, so people with Alzheimer's develop motor problems as well as memory and thinking problems.

One brief note about the latest finding that difficulties with smell (*anosmia*) may be associated with early signs of Alzheimer's disease: The olfactory bulbs (see brain lobes figure below) are located beneath the frontal lobes, and they extend to the deeper structures in the brain, one of which is the hippocampus, which is associated with memory and Alzheimer's. Have you ever smelled something that reminded you of an event or a person? Have you smelled fresh baked bread and immediately felt comforted or happy? This is just another example of how interconnected the brain is and how malfunction in one area (smell) triggers memory and emotion. Understanding this interconnectedness helps us use an impaired sense of smell to find disease in a distant part of the brain, such as the hippocampus. Although those connections exist and are useful for research, the sense of smell deteriorates with age in many people without Alzheimer's, so clinical diagnosis of Alzheimer's on anosmia alone is still not recommended.

The Cortex

You will learn about other subcortical structures as we go on, but first we will discuss the cortex by discussing brain functions and the lobes that are involved. The cortex is divided into four lobes, and this is shown schematically in the next drawing. Each of the four lobes is found in both the left and the right hemisphere. So, for example, there is a left temporal lobe and a right temporal lobe. The four lobes are the frontal, temporal, parietal, and occipital lobes. The next drawing shows a picture of the outside of the brain from the left side. The lobes are labeled.

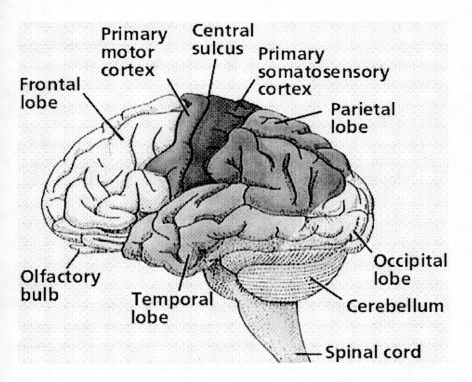

Briefly, the function of the frontal lobe is integration and judgment, the temporal lobes are associated with speech and emotion, the parietal lobes serve to help us determine depth, texture, and other spatial attributes of objects, and the occipital lobes interpret visual information. Just as there is connection between the cortex and the subcortex, and between the right brain and left brain, there is interconnection among the lobes. Remember our basic rule: the brain is highly interconnected. Both the right and left hemispheres of the brain work together to give you the whole picture—the whole perspective. The whole is truly greater than the sum of the parts.

Our brain functions can be divided into several areas: vision, language, memory, executive/motivation, and emotion. To make this easier, we will go function by function and discuss how the brain operates and how dementia can affect that function.

Vision

When we look at an object, its image is converted to chemical impulses in the retina at the back of the eyeball. This information is now in a form that the nerves of the brain can use (See the previous appendix), and the information travels along the nerve cells through the brain to the occipital lobe in the back of the brain. Motion, distance, height, length, shading—all this is conveyed through the neurons in the brain and instantaneously received and interpreted by the occipital lobes. The occipital lobes work in concert with the parietal lobes and parts of the temporal lobes to interpret the visual information and make some sense of it for you. The parietal and temporal lobes are often called the "visual association" area. They process visual information and link it to other brain areas.

When visual information enters the brain through the eyes, the parietal lobes help the occipital lobe to interpret the information by determining angles, depth, texture changes, and spatial relationships. By our ability to recognize faces and objects, we can pick out a friend in a crowd or tell the difference between a baseball bat and a similarly shaped piece of firewood. For example, suppose you are walking down a long hallway carpeted with a dramatic zig-zag pattern of bright contrasting colors. If your occipital and parietal lobes are working normally, you are confident that the floor is always flat, because any changes you see in the texture are related only to color changes. However, if your brain is not working normally, you might think that you are walking on a surface that changes levels or heights or direction. How would you walk on such a surface? Probably, you would walk by holding on to the wall, or as if you were walking on eggshells. You might appear drunk as you tried to navigate your way. You might even lose your balance and fall. Carnival "funhouses" employ the manipulation of the parietal lobe to fool our brains into thinking that surfaces are not what they seem, and we laugh at the way we lurch from safe spot to safe spot, knowing it is all a game.

What if you were a person with dementia and your visual association areas were operating abnormally? It would be like living all the time in one of those "funhouses," except it wouldn't be much fun. This is one reason why people with Alzheimer's disease often appear afraid as they cross a threshold into a new room (especially if the room is dark) or appear unable to "see" handrails tastefully painted the same color as the wall. In assisted living facilities, the tasteful decorating schemes are more often used to provide a "homey" feel, but if colors and textures are too coordinated, the resident with dementia may not be able to find light switches or handrails, or they may not be able to discriminate the closet door from the door to the hallway.

Language

The language association areas are located in the area of the brain where the temporal and parietal lobes adjoin. The left language association area of the brain understands language, both oral and written. In most people who are right handed, the left temporal lobe controls some aspects of speech and language. Without going into too much detail about the process, the temporal lobe allows us to speak in order to express our thoughts. We generate words into meaningful phrases and sentences. Sometimes the first sign of dementia can be problems finding the right words to use when talking, or difficulties coming up with the names of common objects. We all have this problem occasionally, but in Alzheimer's it is to the point that the person has problems communicating with others, and family members are often unable to decipher the message that the affected person is trying to convey. Sometimes the person will use the wrong word for something, resulting in confusion about their message. One family member reported that she had learned to "decode" her father-in-law's communication as his Alzheimer's worsened. Every liquid was called "blood," so he might say, "I want some blood," or "Look out for that blood on the floor." By trying to use context and look at the surroundings, she could determine that he wanted juice, or that he wanted her to avoid the water puddle on the floor. This saved them both a lot of effort and frustration, because she stopped trying to convince him that "blood" was not the correct word to use.

When someone speaks to you or you see written information, you are able to comprehend what you hear or what you read. It is important to realize that although written language is a visual pattern it is comprehended by a different area of the brain than the visual association areas that perceive things and spaces. In other words, language is comprehended by a different area of the brain than the visual association areas that function to perceive things and spaces. People with Alzheimer's will pick up a newspaper and focus their attention on the articles and appear to "read." Families will say to us, "He really enjoys his morning newspaper. He reads every section." However, if you ask the person with Alzheimer's to actually read the words or explain the article or headline, he may not be able to do it, because he cannot interpret the information or recognize the words.

The language association area of the right side of the brain interprets the non-verbal parts of language. That is, various expressions of body language—a gesture, a facial expression, a tone of voice—add meaning to the words someone says. How do you know someone is asking you a question? The voice goes up a little at the end of the sentence, and the person may have raised eyebrows and an expectant look on his face. How do you know what's funny or when someone is kidding around? If someone smiles or laughs, tilts his head back, and slaps his knee, you might think he has made a joke. Rolling his eyes may suggest that someone is being sarcastic. If someone waves at you, you wave back. If they are waving in a rapid manner and they look afraid, you may not wave back, but you may run over to them to see what's wrong. If someone is yelling in an angry way at another person, you understand that he is not angry at you, and you most likely keep your distance from the situation.

If your brain has a disease that interferes with its ability to understand non-verbal messages, you might not know that someone is asking you a question. You might think they are angry, especially if they ask the question in a loud voice. You might not know whether the person who is yelling is mad at you, and you might feel threatened and frightened by them. Teasing and laughing might be misunderstood. A person acting in a hurried manner or using frantic gestures might seem threatening or aggressive to the person with difficulty interpreting non-verbal messages.

Memory

Memory is a very complex and misunderstood function of the brain. Entire volumes of books are dedicated to the topic of memory, and there are a wide variety of memory tests that neuropsychologists use to evaluate how people learn and remember. We know very little about how memories actually get "stored" in our brain cells. We know that emotional reactions, physical conditions like fatigue and illness, and even our own personal biases can affect memory.

Traditionally the temporal lobes of the brain have been associated with memory and emotion. The lobes lie above and next to the subcortical areas that have to do with emotions, body movement, and other automatic functions, as discussed earlier in this appendix. One of the structures that has been clearly associated with memory and with Alzheimer's disease is the hippocampus, which is in the subcortex. If you were to lift up either temporal lobe and look underneath, you would find the hippocampus nestled between that temporal lobe and the deeper structures of the brain. The left temporal lobe is also where verbal memory is managed and supposedly stored. This makes sense, if you consider that it is also where language is processed.

Traditionally, the right temporal lobe is thought to store visual memory. Actually, both temporal lobes act in concert to recall as much information as possible about a stimulus. If you see a picture of a leaf, and you want to remember the picture, it helps to recognize the object, and it also helps to know the name "leaf." However, if there are lots of leaves, then it helps to recall the visual differences between the leaves, rather than just the word "leaf." How might you try to remember the following designs?

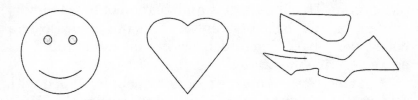

You might think, "smiley face" and "heart" or "valentine" for the first two, but the third figure is not easily recalled just by giving it a name. Instead you must recall the angles and the directions of the lines.

Other structures next to the hippocampus are associated with emotions, which can have great influence on memory. It is clear that we will often remember things better if we have some emotional association to the information. This is a survival skill, because it allows us to remember things that seem dangerous to us, such as the difference between a friend and an enemy. Many people with Alzheimer's will recall the emotional tone of a situation, even when they don't remember the actual details of the event. That is why it is easier for them to remember if they had a good or bad day, rather than what they did all day. Rather than ask what they just ate (What flavor ice cream did you have?), it is easier for them to recall if they enjoyed the time or the food (Did you have fun eating the ice cream?). This "emotional memory," if you will, is also a reason why they may seem afraid or angry at a particular caregiver. Some event or interaction with that caregiver stirs up a memory, but the person with Alzheimer's cannot express to us the details of the event or conversation.

Memory loss is often called "short term memory loss," which means the inability to learn **new** things. Rather than go into details about the varieties of memory processes, for just a minute think of our memory system as a big filing room. This is a **huge** simplification of how memory works, and we beg forgiveness from our neuroscience colleagues. That being said, bear with the humble authors as we describe the brain's "File Room."

Imagine rows upon rows of filing cabinets filled with folders filled with papers. Information or thoughts come into the room as a piece of paper, and the file clerk must store it. Let's say you want to store the name of the hotel where you will stay at a conference this coming October. "Hmm," your filing clerk says as he looks at the writing and the picture, "Hotel Lamont. That would go in the places stayed section, ...Campsites...Bed & Breakfasts... Hotels...ah... October meeting...it goes here." He places the paper in the folder, closes the cabinet, and awaits another piece of paper. Later, when someone asks you where you will be staying for your meeting, the file clerk gets the request, goes to the filing cabinet, pulls open the drawer, looks in the folder, and pulls out the paper. "The Hotel Lamont," you say with confidence as you picture the front of the hotel.

In the filing room of someone with Alzheimer's, the papers with new information don't get filed because folders and filing cabinets are no longer there. Recall from Appendix B that the neurons are frizzled and can't work. Sometimes the papers don't even get to the clerk, or by the time they get to the clerk they have the wrong information on them. The papers pile up, sometimes get thrown away entirely, or are lost. The file clerk can retrieve papers from the few existing file cabinets, because the system is already in place. The file clerk can occasionally find a needed paper in the piles of new information which don't have file cabinets, which is always a big thrill, but he cannot always make any sense of the paper he finds. Eventually the clerk quits, so there is no one left even to retrieve papers filed long ago—important papers like how to chew and swallow. So, that is why a person with memory problems can recall where they grew up, their wedding day, or the name of their best friend in high school, but they cannot recall what they had for breakfast, or whether they ate breakfast.

As we said before, obviously this analogy is very simplistic, but it's still useful. A granddaughter ("Sandy") of a lady with Alzheimer's told us she uses the filing cabinet analogy to reduce her sadness and frustration with her grandmother's memory problems. On one occasion, Sandy had given her grandmother a little ceramic angel to keep on her nightstand. Her grandmother loved angels and seemed to like the gift a lot, and this was important to Sandy. A short time later, when she talked to her grandmother about the angel, grandma could not recall it and said she did not know anything about the angel. Even after Sandy showed her grandmother the angel, the lady was very confused and stated she had never seen it before. This hurt Sandy's feelings, and she began to think her grandmother didn't care. Then she remembered the "filing cabinet" and rather than think her grandmother was ungrateful, told herself that grandmother "just didn't have any filing cabinet for that." The analogy allowed her to put away negative thoughts and objectify her loved one's comments. Now when her grandmother forgets something, Sandy says to herself, "No filing cabinet!" and she is able to move on.

This is not to say before the filing clerk quits that a person with Alzheimer's cannot learn anything. It's just that the learning is typically a very long and difficult process, so it's not reasonable to expect someone with Alzheimer's to learn, "Your daughter will be here in an hour." A person with Alzheimer's can learn routines, as you may have noticed if your loved one in Alzheimer's care knows the times that meals are served. However, part of this is due to the already learned routine of mealtimes over the lifetime. Alzheimer's patients have been known to learn the exit codes for the doors, and to use them when they want to leave. In fact, this is a common problem in dementia care units, which is why we always have to whisper the codes to each other or turn our backs to hide the keypad as we enter the codes to leave the unit.

Memories, especially of well-ingrained routines and activities, will remain. Residents with Alzheimer's will try to leave a facility at the end of the day to "pick up the children from school," or to return home from work. They will see the staff waving, saying goodbye to each other, and leaving, and a memory is recalled, prompting them to want to "go home." They will repeatedly try to pay for meals, even though it is part of the cost of assisted living, because the dining room looks like a restaurant. We are sure you have noticed other behaviors that seem to be like the replaying of old scripts, and now you can understand some of the complex memory work that goes into such behaviors.

Executive Dysfunction

We have discussed the occipital, frontal, and parietal lobes, and now we will discuss one of the most interesting and misunderstood of the lobes: the frontal cortex. When the brain has interpreted what is seen, heard, smelled, tasted, and touched, it communicates with the frontal lobes, which must decide what to do with all that information and direct the action. Our frontal lobes are the "executive" centers. The word "executive", of course, comes from the word "execute." According to Webster's dictionary, execute means "to carry out fully; put completely into effect; to do what is provided or required by." Think about what an executive does in a business. An executive takes in all the interpretations of information and data, puts them in some perspective, and decides what action to take next. Does the CEO form a committee to study the information further? Make an offer to buy? Sell? Hire new people? Ignore the information as unimportant? This is essentially what our frontal lobes do, most of the time without our even realizing how much work is accomplished. They "put completely into effect" the action plan based on all the information they have received. The lobes are in charge of initiation, planning, sequencing, logically reasoning, judging, discriminating appropriate actions from inappropriate actions, and stopping a behavior when the goal is reached. Also, the ability to judge the outcome of our actions helps us to learn from our mistakes and to change our behavior as needed.

Let's say you are sitting in your favorite chair watching television, and you realize you are hungry. There's no one to serve you. What do you do? Well, you probably think about what you might want to eat. Should you prepare something here or get take out? Hot or cold? Meat or no meat? If meat, then what - chicken, beef, pork? How about fish?

Then you may think about what you have in the kitchen to prepare. You have to compare your choices with your inventory. But first, you have the initiative and motivation to get out of your chair and head for the kitchen. Once there, you may open the refrigerator. Where do you look for things? If you decide to have a sandwich, you need to know the inventory of your pantry to determine whether or not you have the ingredients to make the sandwich. Do you have bread? If you don't, you have to change course— can you use a pita? Should you just have tuna salad with no bread? Now you look in the cabinet and decide you may also want chips.

You make your decisions, and you gather all the ingredients. Now you have to put those ingredients all together in at least a reasonable sequence. You get a plate. You get your condiments. The meat and mayonnaise go inside the sandwich, and you have to keep your mind on the sandwich until you finish making it. The telephone may ring, and you need to decide whether to answer it or continue making your lunch. If you answer the phone, you need to persevere and go back and finish the sandwich. You complete making the sandwich, and now you need to decide what to drink.

Is all this sounding too complicated and time consuming? We haven't even examined all the steps in this process, but we can see that even in the steps we have examined, our brains are working furiously. We must focus, plan, sequence, consider consequences, decide on the appropriate action, initiate the appropriate action, and terminate the action when the goal is achieved. While all this is happening, the brain is processing the variety of information that our senses provide us and sending the interpretations to the frontal lobes, which then send it back for more information or to take action.

Disinhibition

Another important role of the frontal lobes is to act as the "hand over the mouth," so we censor ourselves and our behavior. Getting drunk is a very effective way to take the hand away from the mouth and do whatever comes to mind. This one common example of what we call "frontal lobe disinhibition." In other words, the frontal lobes have stopped inhibiting (stopping) someone from engaging in an unacceptable behavior— like dancing around with a lampshade on his head. The frontal lobe functions are the last to develop, and studies report that adolescent frontal lobes are not fully developed. Well, you probably knew that already, but it's good to have some scientific evidence to back up your observations. We all have to learn what actions are acceptable and safe. We learn not to point at people and stare. We learn not to say what we are thinking all the time.

In a person with Alzheimer's disease, the executive control is lost over time. However, executive dysfunction, rather than memory problems, can be one of the earliest signs of dementia. So, the dementia can be missed by others. Consider these situations from the perspective of someone whose brain is impaired from Alzheimer's:

You see person A yelling at person B. If, because of parietal lobe dysfunction, you misperceive that person A is angry (she might just be using a loud voice to be heard), you might feel frightened or threatened. The frontal lobes get that message, and you hit person A. You might try to rescue person B by shoving them out of the way. With a functioning frontal lobe, you would evaluate the situation—perhaps ask person A what is wrong before acting. If, however, you have lost that ability to evaluate and change course, you will simply react.

All too often, we are called by assisted living facilities because someone is "violent," when in reality, that person is simply reacting (without proper frontal lobe function) to a situation. In many cases the environment can be modified rather than using medication to control the behavior. Here's another scenario:

Here's another scenario involving the visual association area function: you see a pretty, young woman (the nurse) who is speaking in a soft, friendly tone of voice. She takes you into the bathroom and starts to unzip your pants (to help you onto the toilet). Your frontal lobes receive the messages without the correct interpretation and context. You believe she likes you and is coming on to you. You reach out to touch her breasts.

Sadly, this is when we get called in to "put an end" to someone's "sexually inappropriate behavior." Often, men are abruptly discharged from facilities because of situations like this, because the caregivers are unaware how the dementia has affected the brain and the inhibitions.

Another important and often overlooked function of the frontal lobes is initiation. Let's return to our sandwich situation and illustrate how impaired frontal lobe function might adversely affect initiation. You are in your favorite chair watching television and you get hungry. You think about what you might want to eat. Your frontal lobes receive more information. You get distracted by the TV show, or by a bird outside the window, or the color of your pants, or the button on your sleeve. The rest of the brain is sending you signals that you cannot ignore or store for later. You continue to sit in your chair for the rest of the day, instead of initiating getting food. Unless assisted living staff are aware of frontal lobe dysfunction in dementia, they are likely to allow you to skip meals, assuming you are not hungry, when, in fact, you simply cannot maintain the focus necessary to get to the dining room to eat.

Perseveration

What if you act on the information you receive but can't stop acting? The following situation is an example of "perseveration," or the inability to stop an activity or shift to the next thing. Ideas or thoughts sometimes don't come to a stop in the brain of a person with Alzheimer's:

You think that you need to check to make sure your

wallet is in your purse. You look through the purse and find your wallet. You look in the wallet and sort the cards and money. You return the wallet to the purse and set it down. Time passes. You think that you need to check to make sure your wallet is in your purse. You look through the purse and find your wallet. You look in the wallet and sort the cards and money. You return the wallet to the purse and set it down. Time passes. You think that you need to check to make sure your wallet is in your purse... etc. etc.

You might think the above situation is just a memory problem, but it's much more complex than that. There is no other activity to distract you, so you keep having the same thought and action repeatedly. A family told us that their father would repeatedly get up from his chair, go to the bathroom to make sure the light was on, and then go sit down for a minute or so. His daughter counted 50 times in a row that he did this. It was not until they had dinner on the table and got him to eat that he stopped the "checking" behavior. The solution, of course, was to interrupt his behavior with some other activity. In the dementia care unit where he lives now, he goes back and forth repeatedly from his room to the nurses' station dozens of times until there is an activity that stops his perseverative behavior.

One of the earliest signs of dementia is this perseveration, and it's often in a form which is quite irritating to family members who don't understand what's happening. Something will happen: for example, the electricity will go off. The person with early dementia might recommend checking the breaker. That is done, the breaker is fine, and it's clear that the entire neighborhood is without electricity. You call the utility company and they report that the line is down, but being worked on.

The person with dementia, although they know that the line is down, continues to suggest checking the breaker. They haven't forgotten the breaker is working, it's just that the response can't be terminated. Family members get annoyed, finally snapping in anger, "Mother, I told you the breaker was fine! Stop asking about it!!" Mother is understandably hurt because she doesn't have the ability to monitor her perseveration and doesn't realize she's doing it—or how annoying she is. She's simply trying to help. You can also see how executive dysfunction alone might appear as if someone is just being "difficult," or "stubborn," or "uninterested," when they are really exhibiting signs of dementia.

"Denial" or Lack of Awareness

One of the hallmarks of Alzheimer's, and the most distressing to families and friends, is the patient's lack of awareness of any cognitive problems. Families will often say to us that their loved one "just doesn't want to admit" there are problems, or they "are afraid to talk about their problems." If you ask someone with Alzheimer's if they have any problems with memory or thinking, they will usually tell you, "No, but my family says I do." It is useless to try to convince them that they have deficits and need help, because the frontal lobes are not working as they should, and therefore, the person has absolutely no awareness of his or her problems. The awareness of one's situation, the implications and the meaning of behavior (our own and others'), are part of what our brain does for us. The ability to judge a situation means that you understand the issues, other people's roles in the situation, how your behavior affects other people, and the possible outcomes of the actions taken.

Because the person with Alzheimer's lacks awareness

that he has a problem, he may interpret events and others' behaviors in a rather bizarre or paranoid way. After all, if you believe your memory is normal, how do you explain that your wallet is not on your dresser? You know you left it there. The only explanation (since you don't realize you have memory problems) is that someone stole it. Someone with Alzheimer's may lose or misplace objects, but they often claim that someone stole them. Sometimes the thinking goes so far as to believe family members or strangers come into their home at night and take valuables. When the objects or valuables are later found, the person with Alzheimer's may attribute this to the perpetrator returning the item because of their conscience, or, even more bizarre, returning an exact replica. (This phenomenon of "delusion of doubles" or duplication with an exact replica has a name: Capgras syndrome, named after the person who first described it.) We have known individuals who claim that family members had come in the night before and moved objects around, such as the mail or a purse, in order to confuse them. This is also why it is difficult for families to try to gain control of the person's finances. If you believe that you are capable of managing your money and you really intend to take care of those bills tomorrow, why would you give up your checkbook to a family member? They may spend all your money—after all, they have been stealing your purse.

Impaired Judgment

If you have Alzheimer's, executive abilities are impaired to the point that judgment is impaired, and you are unable to take appropriate action in situations. So you give the nice man on the phone your social security number because he says he is from the bank, and you believe him. "Oh yes," you will say later, "I know that it's wrong to give out my social security number to just anyone. But he was from the bank. I suppose the people at the bank do call on the telephone. I wouldn't know, I've never worked at a bank." The abstract knowledge of the "correct" thing to do in such a situation is still retained, but the processing and the reasoning in the actual situation is lost. Because executive function is often lost before a person is identified as having dementia, you can see why elders are so vulnerable to exploitation and why public awareness campaigns to "Just Say No" if someone asks you for money will be lost on a person who lacks executive function.

As you can tell by now, basic knowledge of how the brain works is critical to understanding how Alzheimer's affects behavior. Just from reading this and Appendix B, you now know very much more than what is known by almost all caregivers in assisted living and dementia care facilities. Many caregivers, even professional ones, are taught that behavior problems are an inevitable part of the disease process. However, they are not trained why those behaviors occur or which brain function is affected, so they have difficulty interpreting behaviors in such a way that allows them to see patterns and to develop interventions.

LaVergne, TN USA
20 May 2010
183357LV00001B/118/P